The Aging Enterprise

A Critical Examination of Social Policies
and Services for the Aged

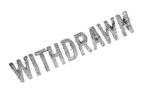

Carroll L. Estes

with contributions by
Philip R. Lee
Lenore Gerard
Maureen Noble

The Aging Enterprise

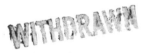

 Jossey-Bass Publishers

San Francisco • Washington • London • 1979

THE AGING ENTERPRISE
A Critical Examination of Social Policies and Services for the Aged
by Carroll L. Estes

Copyright © 1979 by: Jossey-Bass, Inc., Publishers
433 California Street
San Francisco, California 94104
&
Jossey-Bass Limited
28 Banner Street
London EC1Y 8QE

Library of Congress Catalogue Card Number LC 79-83571

International Standard Book Number ISBN 0-87589-410-0

Manufactured in the United States of America

JACKET DESIGN BY WILLI BAUM

FIRST EDITION

Code 7918

The Jossey-Bass
Social and Behavioral Science Series

For my parents, Carroll and Joe Estes,
whose contribution to this endeavor
defies adequate recognition and gratitude.
And for my daughter, Duskie Lynn,
who throughout her short life has
constructed her reality around this research.

Preface

The Aging Enterprise was written because of my strong conviction that present social policies are failing to ameliorate the disadvantaged condition of the elderly in the United States. These policies are failing for many reasons, as I hope to make clear.

I have been involved in aging policy and program issues for more than a decade, as a scholar conducting research and offering testimony before legislative bodies and as a participant observer where I shared the worlds of the individuals and agencies at the center of activities generated by the Older Americans Act. I have also served as a state commissioner on aging, a Gerontological Society officer, and a consultant to the U.S. Senate Special Committee on Aging.

In this book I attempt to illuminate the way we think about the old—and the influence of these dominant attitudes on the larger social, political, and economic elements that have shaped the context of the Older Americans Act and the many other federal policies for the aged. I argue that taken-for-granted assumptions and expectations are at the heart of the social order and that it is crucial to examine them to understand social reality. This application of what sociologists call "the social construction of reality" perspective to the aged is premised on the theory that social and political events, processes, and conditions are the primary determinants of the status of the aged. The added insights of a "political economy" perspective call attention to how social policies and programs for the aged bolster the existing power arrangements of society. Similarly, gerontological theories and social science developments have supported the existing order by overemphasizing research that locates "the problem" within the older individual and his or her aging process, diverting attention away from the social and political production of the problem. These widely held but overindividualized conceptions of the aging problem lead me to argue that because the problems of the aged are neither properly approached nor understood in terms of their structural origins or causation they are not adequately addressed by public policy.

In applying the social construction of reality framework, I have been concerned with delineating the perceptions and interests that shape societal priorities and policies for the old and with the extent to which the elderly influence and benefit from the aging enterprise that has resulted therefrom. In applying the political economy perspective, my concern has been with how social politics for the aged reflect larger political and economic conditions and problems. How groups get what they want and how politics build in the domination of certain special interests over others are among the critical questions I address. My interest has been to analyze these diverse perspectives in a way that is relevant not only to educators, researchers, and practitioners in the field but also to political sociologists, social planners, political scientists, and policy analysts. Policy makers also will find this book of vital interest, and older persons will find many answers to their questions as to why, of all the money allotted for the aged, so little benefit sifts down to them.

The special interests and the government bureaucracies that are aligned with those interests unduly influence the implementation of many federal laws affecting the elderly (for example, Medicare and the Older Americans Act)—primarily because Congress, in enacting the laws, has been intentionally ambiguous in defining the objectives to be achieved as well as the means to achieve them. I hope to demonstrate that legislative encouragement of pluralistic bargaining among the most powerful special interests as the best means for deriving social policy is detrimental to the elderly and to the broader public interest.

The following chapters analyze and assess major legislative enactments for the aged; present a detailed and completely up-to-date examination of the Older Americans Act and existing research concerning implementation of this act; provide an extensive analysis of the problems of accountability and responsiveness attendant to social policies for the aged that embody the new federalism principles of decentralization; and review research on citizen participation and the role of the aged in shaping major federal programs that vitally affect them. The book also describes the interest group politics and intentional ambiguity that characterize and plague such policies and how they provide influence for administering bureaucracies and structurally protected interests.

Social, political, and economic antecedents and consequences of current policies are examined in terms of their symbolic and material benefits for the elderly in the United States; issues of the separatism, stigmatization, and dependency that are fostered by policies for the aged are discussed in the context of the political and economic conditions and problems of the larger society; and the "aging problem" is considered in terms of its political uses and how it serves the expansion of a major industry of aging services.

Increasing attention is being given to the problems of old age—and to the social policies and social costs of this growing segment of the U.S. population. Previous publications on this topic have not combined sociological and political economy approaches to these issues. This book not only explores the origins and consequences of social policies for the aged but also the aging enterprise that has been created by those policies. In the concluding chapter I have attempted to address alternative policy strategies that would require a reconstruction of current social definitions of the problems of old age and the abandonment of the remedies that such definitions now prescribe.

Acknowledgments

The idea for this book was conceived as I was working on my doctoral dissertation, which was funded through a fellowship from the National Institute of Mental Health in 1970 (Grant #SF03-MH4-5336-BEHA). Subsequent support for research on issues related to the Older Americans Act was provided through two general research support grants of the Academic Senate at the University of California, San Francisco, and research funds were made available through the School of Nursing at the same institution. Although not directly supporting the research in this volume, the Administration on Aging is currently providing grant funds for a study of the discretionary policies and funding patterns of state and area agencies on aging (Grant #90-A-979); the conceptualization and design of this research have been instrumental in advancing the ideas presented in this book. The Department of Social and Behavioral Sciences, School of Nursing, at the University of California, San Francisco, graciously permitted me to take my sabbatical at the earliest possible date and provided me with the requisite respite from departmental labor to enable me to finish the writing.

My gratitude extends to many people, for this book is a product of more than ten years of research and academic association. My greatest intellectual debts are to Herbert Blumer, Joseph R. Gusfield, Alvin Gouldner, John Walton, and Randall Collins, each of whom taught me important lessons in sociological criticism, and to Philip Lee, from whom I have gained invaluable understanding of federal policy processes and their consequences. The special concern, colleagueship, and advice which Joseph Gusfield, John Walton, and Philip Lee provided in reading the manuscript must be especially acknowledged, since their thoughtful criticism contributed greatly to the book. My mother, Carroll Cox Estes, an author in her own right, read and reread, edited, and improved every chapter. Anselm Strauss, as my department chair and intellectual colleague, provided support and suggestions.

Many others have contributed significantly to my thinking about the Older Americans Act (some of whom may disagree with my point of view, but all of whom nevertheless were important): William Oriol, staff director of the U.S. Senate Special Committee on Aging, and his staff associate, Kathy Diegnan; Maureen Noble, now a law student at Southern Methodist University, with whom I engaged in a study of paper work and accountability for the Senate Special Committee on Aging; Philip Armour, assistant professor, Department of Social Sciences, University of Texas at Dallas; Betsy Robinson, research associate, and Beverly Edmonds, graduate student and research assistant, Department of Social and Behavioral Sciences, University of California, San Francisco; W. Ray Smith, Administration on Aging Regional Office in San Francisco; Leon Harper, president of the National Association of Area Agencies; and Herman Brotman, winner of the first Kent Award in gerontology. In addition, Robert Benedict (U.S. Commissioner on Aging), Donald Reilley (Deputy Commissioner), Martin Sicker, and Bryon Gold of the Administration on Aging have stimulated my interest and understanding of old age politics from the national scene.

My research staff has made major contributions to the development of this work—often through long hours of discussion and sometimes heated debate. In this process, Robert Newcomer deserves special mention. Not only has he helped sharpen my thinking considerably, but he has admirably and exceptionally kept our research enterprise on target when I was deeply immersed in writing. I also thank Theodore Benjamin, Mollyann Freeman, Mary Kreger, Libby Manthey, Judith Musick, B. J. Curry Spitler, and James Swan. Lenore Gerard provided invaluable editorial assistance as well as legislative research and analysis of particular import to many of the arguments advanced herein. Nancy Brown and Ida Red did a great deal of editorial and bibliographical work. Manuscript coordination and clerical assistance were in the able hands of Maryrose Hendricks, without whose tireless effort this book would never have been completed. Bruce Martin supervised the computerized manuscript preparation, and Alice Rappaport provided emergency clerical assistance. Staff members of the Health Policy Program at the University of California, San Francisco, who spent endless hours in preparing Chapter Six are Nancy Brown (who also provided research assistance), Eunice Chee, Sally Soper, and Barbara Johnson.

I extend a special and personal acknowledgment to my daughter, Duskie Lynn, who not only endured but supported my preoccupation and time commitment to finish "the book." Alicia Martinez provided household continuity. My father Joe Estes gave me, as always, loving support and, together with my mother, assisted in the final weeks of manuscript writing. Last but not least I express my gratitude to Margaret Kuhn, founder and convener of the Gray Panthers, who played a major role in my commitment to the commencement and completion of this work, and to Robert Butler, director of the National Institute on Aging, whose important book, *Why Survive?*, provided inspiration.

None of these individuals, of course, is responsible for the interpretations and commentary in this book.

San Francisco, California   CARROLL L. ESTES
April 1979

Contents

The Author

CARROLL L. ESTES is associate professor of sociology at the University of California, San Francisco, where she teaches courses on medical sociology, political economy, and gerontology and is a faculty member of the graduate program in sociology. She is also a consultant to the U.S. Senate Special Committee on Aging.

Estes was born in Fort Worth, Texas, in 1938; she was awarded the A.B. degree from Stanford University (1959), the M.A. degree from Southern Methodist University (1961), and the Ph.D. degree from the University of California, San Diego (1972)— all in sociology. Her first book, *The Decision-Makers: The Power Structure of Dallas* (1963), received the Matrix Award of the Dallas Chapter of Theta Sigma Phi Journalism Society. Among the other publications she has authored or co-authored are articles in *The Handbook of Aging and the Social Sciences* (with H. E. Freeman, 1976); *Policy Studies Annual Review* (with P. K. Armour and M. Noble, 1978); and articles in *The Gerontologist* (1973, 1976), *The Journal of Gerontology* (1974), *Policy and Politics* (1976), and *Transaction SOCIETY* (1978). She has also co-authored (with M. Noble, 1978)

a report for the U.S. Senate Special Committee on Aging on problems of accountability under the Older Americans Act.

    Estes is now engaged in a major research project, funded
by the Administration on Aging, that focuses on whether decentralization under the Older Americans Act has affected the distribution of services and other benefits to older people; two other
funded research projects pertain to studying the effect of state and
local fiscal problems on health and social services and developing
a data bank of state and local legislative and programmatic innovations in aging for inclusion in the National Clearinghouse on
Aging. Estes is currently working on two other books on "critical
perspectives on gerontology" and the political economy of health
care and is co-directing a training program in applied gerontology.

The Aging Enterprise

A Critical Examination of Social Policies
and Services for the Aged

The Social Construction of Reality: A Framework for Inquiry

====o◻o============o◻o=====

Today there is a cruel and ironic contradiction in the fate of our older citizens. Never before have older people been able to look forward to so many years of vitality. But never before have they been so firmly shouldered out of every significant role in life—in the family, in the world of work, and in the community [Gardner, 1968, p. 153].

The major problems faced by the elderly in the United States are, in large measure, ones that are socially constructed as a result of our conceptions of aging and the aged. What is done for and about the elderly, as well as what we know about them, including knowledge gained from research, are products of our conceptions of aging. In an important sense, then, the major problems faced by the elderly are the ones we create for them.

The lot of these elderly persons, the length and quality of their lives, their participation in community affairs, and their personal levels of gratification are primarily determined by social forces. Although individual differences in such matters as inherited economic status, marital status, and racial and ethnic origins have their influence, the key determinants of the standard of living

1

enjoyed or endured by the aged are national social and economic policies, political decisions at all levels of government, the power of various organized interest groups, and the policies of business and industry.

The policies that social institutions produce reflect the dominance of certain values and normative conceptions of social problems and their remedies. These value choices and definitions of existing conditions are not derived from consensual agreement of the members of society, nor do they result from happy compromises among those persons most affected by them. Some individuals and groups bring greater resources of class, status, and power to influence the definitions of social problems than do others. Although the aged themselves, for example, may attempt to influence socially determined priorities and the resultant public policies, they are only one among a growing number of groups that are vitally interested in determining policy choices on their behalf.

This book is an exploration of what I have called the aging enterprise. This term describes the congeries of programs, organizations, bureaucracies, interest groups, trade associations, providers, industries, and professionals that serve the aged in one capacity or another. Major components include physicians, hospitals, the Social Security Administration, the Administration on Aging, state and area agencies on aging, congressional committees on aging, as well as the nursing home and insurance industries. The aging enterprise includes, but extends far beyond, the so-called aging network—a term coined to describe the many agencies spawned and funded under the Older Americans Act. In using the term *aging enterprise,* I hope to call particular attention to how the aged are often processed and treated as a commodity in our society and to the fact that the age-segregated policies that fuel the aging enterprise are socially divisive "solutions" that single out, stigmatize, and isolate the aged from the rest of society.

Throughout this analysis, the legally mandated organizational caretakers of the problems of the aged are seen as critical in shaping and carrying out public policy. Thus, my concern is largely with organizations, how they function and what roles they play in problem definition and policy formation. The Older Americans Act has been employed as a case study because this enactment is the prototype of public policies affecting the aged. As such, it illustrates how "the problem" has been generally defined and the symbolic manner in which it has been treated. The Older Americans Act illustrates the evolution of public policy and the impact of interest-group politics on that policy—this being typified by the aging network, whose constituent agencies are far more interested in struggling over existing resources than in considering the results of their programs or services. Other important aspects of the Older Americans Act are that it reflects the new federalism principle of decentralization and, as I hope to make clear, the problems of accountability and responsiveness attendant on that policy.

Structure, Ideology, and Paradigm

An examination of the social definitions of aging is important because these definitions are likely to become objective reality in one form or another. It is thus necessary to understand how policies for the aged, and especially those enunciated in the Older Americans Act, contain structural or built-in interests. Applying Alford's (1976) notion of structural interest, one can see that the Older Americans Act institutionalizes the advantages of some selected groups and professions through the structures created in the policy design and implementation requirements of the act. Although there are opportunities for negotiation within the given policy framework, these embedded structural interests limit what the actors in the situation may do. The mandated structural arrangements of agencies and actors that comprise the decision-making network impose limits of choice on both the means and ends, as well as in the negotiation of the implementation processes themselves (Lukes, 1977). In other words, the social structure (as a system of social stratification) delineates the power of individuals and collectivities, as well as the opportunities readily available to them (Twaddle and Hessler, 1977). Opportunities include access to information and the attribution of the prestige and respect that more powerful persons tend to acquire.

Perhaps the most significant aspect of the structural configuration of Older Americans Act policies, and of other aging policies as well, is that they set limits even on what is conceivable

(Lukes, 1977). The perceptions of what is possible become what is real. These "constructions" of reality emerge within the context of legal, economic, and political institutions, which legitimate the dominance of certain interests. They reflect the interests that generate societal consensus, conferring power on some and not on other interests. The result is that the aged, indeed all of us, "come to accept as inevitable that which exists and even believe that it is right" (Alford, 1976, p. 7).

But structural interests are not the only determinants of social policy: ideologies also exert a powerful influence. Bailey describes an ideology as "an organized set of convictions . . . which enforces inevitable value judgements" (1975, p. 32). What is important about ideologies is that they reflect the social position and socially determined values of their beholders and are only partial perspectives. Historically, the notion of ideology has referred largely to the class basis of ideation (Marx [1867], 1961). As belief systems, ideologies are world views competing for definition; and they hold major implications for power relations, for in enforcing certain definitions of the situation, they have the power to compel certain types of action while limiting others. For us, the challenge is to make explicit how certain ways of thinking about the aged as a social problem (and the logical extension of these views into social policies) are rooted in the structure of social and power relations and how they reflect and bolster the social location of their adherents and proponents.

One prominent ideology in American society defines old age as a problem characterized by special needs that require special policies and programs. This belief supports governmental interventions that separate the aged from the rest of society. This belief has had a powerful and pervasive influence on public policies for the aged. The second ideology fosters the belief that the democratic process is synonymous with interest-group bargaining and that the public interest is adequately represented in such processes. This belief system, in turn, justifies the determination of social policies for the aged largely as a consequence of interest-group accommodation among the agencies and professionals that make up the aging network. These two ideologies—separatism and pluralism—are at the core of American social policy for the aged, and they are two of the important themes that will be fleshed out later in this book.

Almost as important as ideology have been the paradigms used to define the problems of the elderly and specific solutions for them within the framework of federal policies, including the Older Americans Act. The impact of a dominant paradigm on perception is "one of reality definition" (Rose, 1971, p. 21), and provides a recipe that makes the problem routine by explaining it (Berger and Luckmann, 1966). Paradigms are the coherent frameworks in which disparate facts are ordered and related. As applied to social policies, the principal function of paradigms is to guide policy construction by organizing certain facts into causal theories that then specify appropriate policy interventions. Because they include problem definitions and the ordering of what is considered relevant and valid knowledge, paradigms limit intervention choices by systematically excluding consideration of alternative frameworks (or interventions). Paradigms themselves may take on the character of ideologies as well as reflect ideologies.

As defined in the Older Americans Act, the problem of the aged is seen as primarily one of fragmentation of services. The paradigm implicit in this problem definition limits the scope of intervention efforts and results in an emphasis on planning, coordination, and pooling of resources to create comprehensive service systems as the major solution. The vagueness and ambiguity implicit in such terms as *planning* and *pooling* has given different interest groups and professionals the opportunity to redefine the solution as falling within their own special domains of responsibility. In this process, the aged are perceived as dependent and in need of the special services prescribed and provided (largely) by these professionals.

Existing institutional and power relationships are maintained by a policy paradigm that imposes problem definitions that in turn legitimate the rationalization (through planning) and reorganization (through coordination) of existing services. The inherent contradiction of such a paradigm is that it cannot solve the problems of the aged because it never addresses them. The vague mandates, constricted programs, and measured appropriations of the Older Americans Act have resulted in services that reach only a small percentage of the elderly. The contrast between the sweeping objectives of the Older Americans Act and the limited authority provided to the Administration on Aging and other agencies created and supported under the act points to the symbolic nature of the act. This symbolism is not inconsequential, however, in that it generates rising expectations and demands, thereby expanding the resource base of organizational service providers, while simultaneously confusing the public and, most importantly, the aged themselves as to the realistic potential for American social policy to alter their social status and improve their condition.

The Social Construction of Reality

For the past thirty years research on the problems of the aged has focused largely on the individual and the adjustment of the individual to circumstances that for the most part were externally determined (Estes and Freeman, 1976; Freeman, 1978). Equally important has been the interpretation of research results. Knowledge is socially generated; it emerges from the ordering and interpretation of facts. It may be accepted as factually legitimate, based upon empirical demonstrations of proof or upon the judgments of proclaimed experts and authorities who possess status and power. The less the knowledge base is empirically proven, the greater the influence of social and political factors in the interpretation and acceptance of data as knowledge.

As definitions of reality become widely shared, they are institutionalized as part of the "collective stock of knowledge" (Berger and Luckmann, 1966, p. 67). Although socially generated, such knowledge and expert opinion take on the character of objective reality, regardless of inherent validity. This "knowledge," in turn, heavily influences both the perception of social problems and ideas on how to deal with them. It is in this sense that the aged have only the social problems that have been "given" them by society. Thus, social researchers and others involved in the design and implementation of intervention programs are not neutral in their influence. "Rather, they are actively engaged in modifying and structuring social reality for the aged" (Estes and Freeman, 1976, p. 539).

Theories of Aging. Although empirical research in aging provides a partial basis for policy development, even more important is the potential contribution of gerontological theory to the underlying rationale for those policies. Because social scientists, as well as policy makers and other elites, contribute to social constructions of reality, the production of gerontological knowledge and its role in public policies deserves careful study—particularly in light of the sociological observation that empirical and theoretical advances occur as a consequence of the interaction between (1) technical development and elaboration (research methodologies, empirical findings, and knowledge) and (2) extratechnical sources, such as changes in sentiments, in background assumptions, and in the personal realities of scientists and those around them (Gouldner, 1970). This central point, that there are nonobjective social and political bases to development of knowledge and ideas, should be kept in mind as we discuss some prominent theories in aging because the ideas advanced in these theories may shape or justify social policies for the aged.

Since the early 1960s, four major social theories of aging have emerged. In order of their development, they are: (1) disengagement theory, (2) activity theory, (3) developmental theory, and (4) symbolic interactionist theory. Disengagement theory (Cumming and Henry, 1961; Cumming, 1974; Henry, 1964) postulates the mutual withdrawal of the aging individual and society. Described as intrinsic to the process of aging and beneficial for both society and the aged individual, disengagement theoretically functions to prepare society for the replacement of its members when they die. At the same time, this process is said to assist the individual in preparing for his or her own death (Cumming and Henry, 1961).

Disengagement theory emerged from the findings of a study of healthy, white, middle-class Kansans—some middle aged and others elderly—many of whom reported that role disengagement did not impair, but rather enhanced, their lives (Cumming and Henry, 1961). While subsequent research has studied the engagement, morale, integration, and activity of individual older persons, the societal aspect of the theory, why and how society withdraws from the aged and with what consequences, has not been empirically studied; rather, societal disengagement is treated as intrinsic, nonproblematic, and beneficial—mandatory retirement (Cohen, 1976) and other government policies that encourage disengagement by restricting the involvement of older persons in society illustrate this. Perhaps most important, this theory provides a rationale for excluding the elderly from the mainstream of society by arguing that mutual withdrawal benefits both the individual and society and that society should not intervene in the aging process and thereby inhibit the natural disengagement of the individual from society. Social services, if provided at all, should not seek to revitalize the aged. Instead, the withdrawal of the individual from society should be encouraged.

In contrast to disengagement theory, activity theory holds that high levels of social activity result in high morale and life satisfaction (Havighurst, 1963). Activity is proposed as essential to successful aging, as is the maintenance of one's middle-age activity patterns (Schooler and Estes, 1972). Lost social roles must be replaced by substitute roles and activities. One implication of the theory is that, to be adjusted, older people must deny the existence of old age by maintaining middle-age life-styles as long as possible. The theory views older people as aging successfully if they continue (or replace) their social involvement. It calls for policies that address socialization and social integration and suggests such social activities for the aged as recreation programs.

The developmental or life-cycle theory stresses the psychological or personality aspects of the aging process. One of its basic tenets is that persons, young and old, are not alike and have their own personalities and styles of living (Neugarten and others, 1964; Lowenthal, 1975). An individual is said to age successfully if he or she maintains a mature, integrated personality while growing old. This is the basis of life satisfaction (Neugarten, Havighurst, and Tobin, 1963). Successful aging is not determined by common normative standards; one provides one's own standards. Some adherents of the theory argue that with age, individuals gain a greater sense of freedom to do what they want, while caring less about what others think. Therefore, there are many ways of growing old, just as there are many ways of becoming adolescent or middle aged. Policy based on developmental theory could rationalize the continuance of laissez-faire approaches to problem solving. A logical extension of this idea might be that concerted policy interventions are unnecessary or not feasible because of the multiple variations in the aging processes of different individuals.

Finally, the symbolic interactionist view of aging, which takes empirical support from a number of studies (Rose and Peterson, 1965; Trela, 1971), argues that it is possible for the interactional context and process (the environment, the persons, and encounters in it) to significantly affect the kind of aging process a person will experience (Gubrium, 1973); changes in the interactional variables may produce results that are erroneously attributed to inherent maturational changes. Disengagement, low self-esteem, and dissatisfaction are seen as resulting from the interpretations and meanings generated in encounters between the aged and others. Both the self and society are seen as capable of creating new alternatives. Social context is crucial; cultural meanings and values are critical and dynamic rather than universal or unchanging. The symbolic interactionist perspective emphasizes the diversity of outcomes that can result from variations in individual commitments and the salience of different issues and situations to the participants (Hall, 1973). For example, individuals of different social, economic, and racial backgrounds have different interests that may affect how they experience and react to aging.

Policies based on the symbolic interactionist framework take an optimistic view of the aged. This theory does not identify particular behavior, activity patterns, or experiences with old age but rather emphasizes the social construction of these in light of interpreted and negotiated interactional encounters. Because symbolic interactionism focuses on both environment and individual, one policy emphasis might be on interventions that seek to modify environmental constraints (for example, the elimination of age discrimination in employment) and another on those directed to the needs of the individual, such as Medicare.

Each of these theories has been criticized on theoretical and methodological grounds, and their empirical support is either weak or incomplete. Disengagement theory is criticized, first of all, as erroneously attributing to intrinsic aging processes phenomena that are also a consequence of the social and normative aspects of aging (Maddox, 1972; Hochschild, 1975; 1976). On an empirical level, Tallmer and Kutner (1969) found no relationship between age and disengagement when they controlled for involuntary role loss of widowhood, retirement, and poor health. Havighurst (1963) and Neugarten, Havighurst, and Tobin (1963) found little evidence of high morale or life satisfaction when disengagement through role loss occurs. Differences in environmental opportunities produce different patterns of engagement and disengagement among the aged (Carp, 1968). These and other findings (Roman and Taietz, 1967) tend to support Hochschild's (1975, 1976) and Cutler's (1976) contention that the "opportunity structures" for participation, and other nonchronological, social aspects of aging, are crucial in explaining engagement/disengagement patterns of older persons.

Activity theory is criticized because "it says nothing about what happens to people who cannot maintain the standards of middle age" (Atchley, 1972, p. 35). Data have been accumulated that contradict activity theory: some older persons are passive, disengaged, and happy; others maintain high activity levels and are not happy. Activity theory is criticized for inattentiveness to contingencies in the larger social environment (social structure, historical context, interactional encounters and opportunities) that condition activity patterns in old age. Data indicate that active people have better physical and mental health and take greater satisfaction in life than do the inactive. It has been demonstrated, however, that such people are better educated and have more money and alternatives than those who are less active. It is not possible at present to distinguish generational from maturational variables in the association between activity, on the one hand, and life satisfaction, health, and well-being, on the other, nor is there certainty about which is cause and which effect.

The complexity of the developmental theory, which states that "there are literally hundreds of possible combinations of reactions to aging" (Atchley, 1972, p. 36), makes it difficult to test methodologically because it posits that an individual's reaction to aging is explained through the interrelationships among biological and psychological changes, the continuance of lifelong patterns, social opportunities, and so forth. It focuses primarily on the individual as the unit of analysis, and little emphasis is given to the role of external social factors per se in modifying the aging process.

Symbolic interactionism has been criticized for minimizing the social and structural constraints that impede interactional opportunities and affect the content of interactional communication. Class differences, for example, restrict the range and content of possible social encounters; all participants do not equally influence the encounter (Lichtman, 1970; Mueller, 1973; Colfax and Roach, 1971). These criticisms may be incorrect or premature, however, since the theory does not inherently ignore the impact of social class and other status and structural factors on aging (Hall, 1973). Nevertheless, with few exceptions (Rose and Peterson, 1965; Hall, 1973) interactionist studies have not been concerned with such issues of power.

At best, the utility of disengagement, activity, and life-cycle theories in advancing our understanding of the aging process is limited. At worst, these theories negatively affect the development of public policies for the aged. As methodologically and empirically employed to date, none of the three theories takes a direct interest in the social structure and the cultural and historical contexts in which the aging process occurs, although lip service is often given to the importance of these factors (Maddox, 1972; Hochschild, 1975). As a consequence, the effects of social conditions, social class, sex, and ethnic differences are largely ignored or unexplored, as are the consequences of institutional racism, sexism, and agism as they differentially influence the aging experience. Symbolic interactionist theory considers these factors, but insufficient empirical study has been carried out to draw more than tentative conclusions that might have policy relevance. One strength of the interactionist inquiry is its concern with the meanings that actors attach to what they do and experience. Such differential meanings provide a basis for assessing whether young and old can find common ground for approaching the problems generated in old age and the potential for political mobilization on old age policy issues. Nevertheless, none of these theoretical approaches has accorded sufficient attention to the social, economic, and political conditions that dramatically affect not only the elderly but those of all ages. The inadequacy of much of the research on old age comes from its focus on what old people do rather than on the social conditions and policies that cause them to act as they do (Estes, 1978). What, for example, is the relationship between the unemployment problems of the elderly and the larger economic problems of capital accumulation? Lacking a sociology of knowledge, gerontology has not examined the technical and extratechnical sources (and consequences) of the perceptions of old age and the labeling of this social problem by "experts," including social scientists.

The central themes in American social gerontology have been concerned with the psychological and social-psychological processes of aging, focusing largely on *individuals* (Marshall and Tindale, 1975; Estes and Freeman, 1976). Little research has been devoted either to person/collectivity/environment interactions and mediations that constrain (or expand) the possible experiential, behavioral, and societal outcomes of old age or to the concerns of a political economy perspective. At the same time, the dominance of psychological testing and other positivistic research methodologies inherited from the initial discipline in social gerontology (psychology) has limited the legitimacy accorded to in-depth observational approaches and has discouraged trust in, and researcher reliance upon, the perspectives and meanings generated and expressed by older persons themselves. Thus, the more problematic and devastating aspects of aging and its variability have been too little emphasized and studied. In addition, political science and sociological concerns with democratic participation in the 1950s fostered an emphasis on individual, social, and political participation, particularly in its most legitimate and formal forms, such as voting and voluntary association membership. These perspectives had a significant impact on the developing field of gerontology. Far less attention has been accorded the larger socio-political conditions that generate the necessity for social policies for such groups as the elderly. Still in its early stage, gerontology has itself shown little interest in the social and political components of its developing knowledge base, and it is characterized by nonreflexive approaches that protect and insulate researchers from "hostile" information (Gouldner, 1970).

Labeling the Problem. One major effect of these theoretical perceptions of aging as a social problem has been the labeling of the aged. Becker (1963) and Matza (1969) have examined the social determinants and consequences of deviant labels and the effects of such labels on the persons to whom they are applied. Labeling theory holds that neither a social problem nor deviance is inherent; rather, they reside in the *reactions* that others have to a situation or an individual. The designation of a social problem "depends on how other people react to it" (Becker, 1963, p. 11). Deviance "is created by society . . . by making the rules whose infraction constitutes deviance . . . . The deviant is one to whom that label has successfully been applied" (p. 87). From this perspective, aging becomes a social problem only when it is successfully labeled as such by some social group. Further, the more influential the group doing the labeling, the more widespread the acceptance of the label. A form of power thus accrues to those politicians, policy makers, administrators, practitioners, and researchers who construct the versions of reality that then determine social policies and intervention strategies.

A potentially important source of power also resides in the *consequences* of these perceptions of reality for the persons so labeled, in this instance, the elderly. Symbolic interactionists tell us that, in developing our own self-concept, we learn to view ourselves in part by reflecting back on our behavior from the point of view of other people (Mead, 1934; Blumer, 1969). Thus, one consequence of labeling may be to alter a person's self-image in a positive or negative direction, depending upon how others look upon and label him (Scott, 1970). This creates a looking-glass self wherein the perception of something as real makes it real in its consequences (Thomas, 1970). Stereotypes of old persons as senile and sexless may *teach* older persons that they are becoming senile and sexless so that they act the part, irrespective of their competence and sexual potency. This is sociogenic aging—"the role which society imposes on people as they reach a certain chronological age" (Comfort, 1976b, p. 9). Older persons, like everyone else, operate from a premise of meanings derived from, and modified on the basis of, the interactions they have with others in their environment. If, in these interactions, old people encounter negative perceptions and labels, they are likely to come to share similar negative perceptions both of themselves and of other older persons.

Such constructions or definitions of reality obviously have political ramifications. They can be translated into public policy decisions affecting resource allocations, and they can come to be

shared by the general public and influence the way in which
younger members of society interact with older persons. As a consequence of their claim to knowledge and expertise, professionals
and practitioners working in gerontology influence conceptions of
problems and solutions at official levels of government. These
views of reality constructed by experts and institutionized by public
policy have profound political and social consequences for the
aged. As the dominant views of the experts come to be accepted
by policy makers, the aged have less and less power to alter the
situation. As Comfort describes it: " 'Oldness' is a political institution and a social convention based on a system which expels people . . . . [It] is a political transformation which is laid upon you
after a set number of years, and the ways of dealing with it are
political and attitudinal" (1976b, p. 28).

This book explores the problems of the elderly from the
basic premise that reality is socially constructed and that these constructions take on an objective quality because people act as if they
point to concrete realities. This is not to assert that the elderly face
no problems independent of those that are perceived as real.
There are, indeed, phenomena associated with chronological aging
and structural conditions that may be said to be objectively real,
regardless of how they are perceived. Social action, however, is in-
divisible from the socially constructed ideas that define and provide images of these phenomena. These ideas, in turn, are affected
by the dominant ideologies and paradigms, as well as by the organizational and interorganizational political resources of interest
groups and advocacy organizations for the elderly, all of which
bear upon the definitions of social problems and their prescribed
solutions.

The social construction of reality perspective provides several useful insights: The experience of old age is dependent in
large part upon how others react to the aged; that is, social context
and cultural meanings are important. Meanings are crucial in influencing how growing old is experienced by the aging in any given
society; these meanings are shaped through interaction of the aged
with the individuals, organizations, and institutions that comprise
the social context. Social context, however, incorporates not only
situational events and interactional opportunities but also struc-

tural contraints that limit the range of possible interaction and the degree of understanding, reinforcing certain lines of action while barring others.

Older persons individually are powerless to alter their social status and condition because their problems and appropriate remedies are socially defined, largely by the dominant members of the society. Since the labels and definitions applied to any group in society result from reciprocal relationships in which the relative power, class, and social standing of interactants play a part, the aged cannot unilaterally alter their relationship to the rest of society.

II

Old Age and the Services Strategy: A Political Economy Perspective

═══════════○▭○═══════════○▭○═══════════

Throughout history, the class struggle governs the manner in which old age takes hold. . . . The meaning or lack of meaning that old age takes on in any given society puts the whole society to the test, since it reveals the meaning or lack of meaning of the entirety of life [de Beauvoir, 1972, p. 10].

Old age in America is viewed as a problem. Common knowledge, political language, social values, and public policies reflect this fact. The political, economic, and social consequences of this widely held belief result from defining the problem of old age as: (1) special and different from others in society and thus requiring special treatment; (2) characterized by an inevitable physical decline of the individual that justifies the stigmatization and continuing marginality of the aged; (3) comprised of a divisible set of needs that can be converted into commodities or services for consumption by the aged; (4) remediable largely through national policies focused on the social integration and socialization of the elderly (rather than policies that would address the disadvantaged status of the aged and thus might improve their social and economic status); and

16

(5) having reached crisis proportions, justifying policies and the expenditure of funds to expand the service economy.

As noted in Chapter One, a pervasive and powerful American ideology sets the aged apart from the rest of society as a group with needs that require special policies and programs. The adoption of this ideology has been deemed necessary by the most sincere advocates for the aged, but its application has been at the expense of the aged themselves. This approach institutionalizes and reinforces the marginality of the aged by legitimating an industry of agencies, providers, and planners that must then continually reaffirm the outgroup status of the aged in order to maintain and expand their own activities. These special policies and programs segregate and stigmatize the aged, although theoretically they exist for the purpose of securing for the elderly a fair share of available resources. Policies limited to particular age clienteles foster an age-segregated society. They are likely to promote divisiveness and conflict among age groups in struggles for scarce resources. They engender competition among these groups and encourage the notion that there can be no equity, just trade-offs. They create simplistic but dangerous dichotomies, such as the young versus the old and the poor versus the middle class. Such policies do not advance society or the cause of social justice, but rather they perpetuate acceptance of the status quo and the inevitability of scarcity, inequity, and intergroup rivalries.

The stigmatization of the aged may also cause them to be seen as responsible for their own problems and therefore undeserving of public action to ameliorate their disadvantaged status. While separatist thinking is strongly contested by such activist groups as the Gray Panthers, it is supported by many providers, including those who stand to benefit by the further entrenchment of pluralistic market approaches to services that assure costly, often profit-making, fragmentation. Recent federal initiatives emphasizing the frail elderly as a priority group for Older Americans Act services lend support to the decremental/decline notion of aging, just as an emphasis on the pervasiveness of disability and chronic illness provides the rationale for these policies. The decremental focus also encourages policies that apply equally to all social classes, while ignoring less popular programs that might highlight the poverty status of the aged. This classless view of aging emphasizes the similarities (and negative image) of all older persons: everybody, no matter what his or her social class, ages physiologically. De-emphasized are the differences across sex, ethnic, and class boundaries within the same age group.

The concept of the aged as dependent and in need of help fosters services strategies that focus on "alleviation of deficient behaviors, not on enrichment or prevention" (Baltes, 1973). Such policies also function as social control mechanisms insofar as they provide an example to the less fortunate members of society of all ages that there will be no relief provided for the aged and they must discipline themselves to work hard and dutifully save, lest they face a deservedly impoverished old age. For the poor and the middle class the message is that they must try harder. If they do not achieve security, it is their own fault. Thus, public policies that tend to maintain the status quo receive support, while those that would redistribute income or other resources to a significant extent are not considered politically feasible. Medicare and the Older Americans Act are two examples of policies that focus primarily on individuals and do little to alter their basic condition or status in society.

Medicare was originally meant to eliminate the financial barriers to medical care for the aged, to provide access to mainstream medical care, and to remove the specter of catastrophically expensive illness from the aged. But it was deliberately designed to avoid modification of the fee-for-services system that is the basis of American medical care. As a result, inflation in the cost of medical care, due primarily to extraordinary price increases for hospital and physician services, as well as to the uncontrolled application of technology in medical care, has virtually eliminated the early gains for the elderly. The aged now pay more out of pocket for their medical care than they did prior to the enactment of Medicare in 1965, and many have had to limit their use of services or turn to the government for additional financial aid through Medicaid, a federally assisted, state-administered program designed to pay for medical care for the poor. Further complicating the aged's access to care is the fact that many physicians no longer accept Medicare reimbursement for their services, preferring instead to charge the patient directly in order to collect higher fees. Even more physicians do not accept any patients, including the aged, whose care is paid for in whole or in part by Medicaid. Thus, the promise of mainstream medical care is a hollow one for millions of elderly who continue to rely on public hospitals and other municipal health services. This focus on the needs of the aged, rather than on the defects of the medical care system, has proved costly for the aged, as well as for the general public (U.S. Senate, 1978b). With emphasis on the individual and fee-for-service treatment, insufficient attention is given to the organization and financing of health care. For the aged, there have been out-of-pocket medical expenses; for the public, there have been highly inflationary and escalating health care costs.

The service strategy of the Older Americans Act assumes that the aged will ultimately benefit from planning, coordination, and the elimination of service fragmentation. This act inserts the professional perspectives and interests of planners and providers between the problems experienced by the aged (often generated by society) and the amelioration of those problems, and it proposes that the appropriate intervention strategy is planning-coordination-bureaucratic reform, not structural reforms that might threaten the beneficiaries of current political and economic arrangements. While the Older Americans Act emphasizes the need to secure dignity, social integration, and independence for the aged, its implementation fosters a separate network of services (meals, recreation, transportation) that isolates the elderly from the American mainstream and other age groups.

The prescribed policy solutions to the problems of the aged, then, take many forms, ranging from the services strategy of the Older Americans Act to the payment for medical care established by Medicare. No matter what the form, however, governmental assistance is offered in ways that foster two types of social control over the aged (Ehrenreich and Ehrenreich, 1974): First, the more advantaged aged are symbolically bought off (co-opted) with direct services and policies that are not limited to the low-income elderly and that focus on their social integration and adjustment through recreational and socialization services—for example, the meals program of the Older Americans Act, whose goal of socialization is at least as important as its nutrition goal. The lack of need-based barriers to services encourages the middle-class elderly to enter service recipient roles, and sympathetic treatment may well render them vulnerable to professional management of an increasingly large part of their lives. Secondly, disciplinary social control is achieved through policies that do nothing to relieve the condition of poverty that faces nearly one third of all the aged and more than one third of the minority and female aged (U.S. Senate, 1978b). Such policies instruct middle- and lower-income Americans in the ethos of hard work based on fears of economic insecurity (O'Connor, 1973) and of their potential impoverishment in old age. These fears keep many working despite onerous conditions and low wages.

The Political Economy and the Definition
of the Problems of the Aged

Political and economic conditions affect how social problems, including the problems of the aged, are defined and treated (Miller, 1976, p. 138). Or, to put it more directly, the state of the economy influences social policies. For example, when the economy is expanding, optimism abounds and resources for dealing with social problems are likely to increase. Conversely, in times of economic restraint, less costly, limited, and in fact inadequate social programs tend to be produced, and their predictable failure then provides a rationale for debunking efforts at social change and for limiting additional resource investments for the disadvantaged. Such government policy contractions occur precisely when the disadvantaged are hardest hit by the same deteriorating economic conditions that foster the retrenchment policies.

Definitions of the social problem of aging and of solutions in the form of policies and programs have reflected the ups and downs of the American economy and shifting bases of political power during the past twenty years. After the economic rebound from the recession of the late 1950s, there was a period of rapid economic growth and political optimism in dealing with the two most difficult domestic social problems—racial discrimination and poverty. This optimism is reflected in the activity theory of aging (socialization and recreation) and was based on the assumption that health, mobility, adjustment, and general well-being are realistic outcomes for most older Americans. This optimism was also evident in the enactment of Medicare, which was to provide all of the elderly with adequate medical services.

Thus, in the 1960s the initial policy of treating the aged as a homogeneous category was established. All aged were lumped together as a general social class with little specificity as to whether they were disadvantaged or how class, race, sex, or ethnic differences affected their status. The Older American Act envisioned the core problems of the elderly as social isolation and the lack of social activity. Hardship differences among the aged were underplayed in favor of social and recreational programs for which all the aged were eligible. These approaches eradicated the visibility of the elderly who were poor, extremely disabled, or ill. The predominantly recreational programs for the aged of the 1960s occurred within the context of the New Frontier and Great Society programs for youth, which were predicated on the assumption that social problems were soluble if only the correct techniques were applied (for example, economic expansion, rational planning, or broadened civic participation). As economic growth and the Vietnam War fueled inflation, the optimism of the 1960s was replaced by disillusionment. The ensuing economic fallout of recession and near depression, coupled with continued inflation, engendered the move for retrenchment of federal programs in the 1970s under the name of decentralization.

The consequence has been to shift responsibility for priorities and dollar decisions, as well as pressures for increased support, from federal to state and local governments, or, as in the case of Medicare, increasingly to the beneficiaries, who must pay higher and higher health insurance premiums and whose out-of-pocket costs continue to grow rapidly. In the early 1970s, policies and programs for the aged emphasized coordination, planning, and comprehensive service development, with only the remnants of a citizen participation strategy and little attention to low-income and minority aged. The 1973 amendments to the Older Americans Act created substate planning/coordinating bodies called area agencies on aging and assigned them responsibility for pooling resources.

It was hoped that this strategy would curtail the growth of federal resource commitments by decentralizing both the focus of demand and the burden for program development and support.

Social policies based on the assumption that the problems of the aging result from the fragmentation of services and necessitate a planning/coordination strategy ignore the widespread poverty of the aged and provide no direct economic relief. Instead the aged become consumers of services that simply feed the expanding service economy. In this sense, the Older Americans Act amendments confirm Miller's (1976) thesis that the treatment of social problems during the 1970s mirrors the central task of the decade—to put the economy on its feet. This notion, that "the business of America is business," emerges periodically as a major theme of public policy. The current emphasis by the Carter administration on the role of the private sector in dealing with major social problems is merely the most recent reflection of this approach. Under such conditions, policy makers tend to take a conservative "reaction" approach to social problems rather than the "action" approach of the 1960s. The 1970s look upon social problems as intractable and thus not remediable by government intervention. This, in turn, justifies the reduction of social programs and the emphasis on the role of the private sector in dealing with problems.

If inflation and a no-growth economy persist, social problem definitions and social policies will increasingly reflect these conditions. Continuation of the current fiscal crisis, both in America and worldwide, will likely engender a lowering of public expenditures for welfare programs in the face of strong counterpressures to protect individual spending power by maintaining current levels of personal disposable income (Abel-Smith, 1978). Hence, social problems of the aged in the late 1970s and into the 1980s will probably be defined in terms of an orientation with disengagement theory that is geared toward individual pathologies and the functional incapacity of the aged. This would be consistent with the return to policy trends that emphasize individual responsibility and productivity. The 1978 Older Americans Act reauthorization includes, for example, a mandate for the Administration on Aging to develop and demonstrate long-term care services. The growing concern with the elderly who are in frail health also reflects this shift in emphasis—to label aging as primarily a problem of personal functioning is to deny recognition of the aggregate marginal economic and social status of the aged, while drawing attention to individual problems. Such a reorientation provides the necessary market development for an expanded service economy (probably in the private sector), consonant with O'Connor's (1973) prediction that a social industrial complex may develop in the United States in response to the growing fiscal crisis. At the same time, such policies demonstrate political responsiveness to the anticipated demographic explosion of the elderly and their growing political organization.

In the early 1960s it was recognized that the aged represented a market for service providers and that there was ample opportunity for business expansion in such areas as hospital construction and drugs. In 1963 Congressman John Fogarty, the acknowledged "Mr. Health" of the U.S. House of Representatives, said of the aged: "I might add in passing that this group represents a $35 billion a year market in the United States and that 17 out of every 100 eligible voters in the United States are over 65" (U.S. House, 1963, p. 10).

In the decade after Mr. Fogarty's remarks, the health industry became acutely aware of the potential market for individual services that older people represented. Surgical services, inpatient hospital care, and prescription drugs for the elderly increased dramatically after Medicare was enacted. All of these services, it should be noted, are physician, not patient, initiated. Over one million workers were added to the health care industry, largely to expand inpatient hospital and nursing home care in response to the demand generated by Medicare and Medicaid. In the decade from 1966 to 1976 the total amount spent on medical care for the aged rose at an average annual rate of 15.5 percent, from $8.2 billion in 1966 to $34.9 billion in 1976. The bulk of the funds went for inpatient care. In 1966, 40 percent of the money went to hospitals and 15 percent went to nursing homes. By 1976, hospitals were receiving 45 percent and nursing homes 23 percent, for a total of 68 percent of all money spent on medical care for the aged. These increased expenditures contributed significantly to the growth of the hospital and nursing home industries. Home health services, largely serving the elderly, also expanded rapidly during this period. The potential for future expansion of services for the aged is great because of the growth of the population aged sixty-five and over, particularly those aged seventy-five and over.

Unilateral Dependency

The expansion of services for the aged is not without consequences. The dominant response to the problems of social groups that are defined as "deviant" by those who hold power has been to establish bureaucratic structures to deal with them. Such structures, and the middle-class bureaucrats by whom services usually are delivered, are the medium for interaction between members of lower social classes and the general society. As described by Sjoberg, Brymer and Farris (1966), the dominant characteristics of such interactions tend to be confusion on the part of some clients and manipulation of the system by others. Certain classes of clients are better able to manipulate bureaucracy than others, while lower-class clients have been found to be at a distinct disadvantage when dealing with bureaucracies, partly because of the application of formal rules and regulations to them and partly because of the ease with which bureaucrats can maintain social distance from them. In this way, bureaucracies tend to "reinforce the class structure" (Sjoberg, Brymer, and Farris, 1966, p. 326).

Under the Older Americans Act the comprehensive planning and services strategies attempt to meet the needs of the poor through imposition of bureaucratic and professional norms. The prescribed solutions to the needs of the elderly fall into several broad service categories—area planning and social services, multipurpose senior centers, and nutrition and employment programs. In general, these services strategies assign to the aged a dependent status and give them little opportunity to reciprocate for services received. In an achievement-oriented society this kind of unilateral dependence is likely to result in a lowered social status for the recipients of services. Simply stated, the notion of welfare assistance implies taking from the rich and giving to the poor. However, instead of reducing differences between rich and poor, such assistance "accepts and bolsters them" (Coser, 1963, p. 148) by institutionalizing the differences.

The services strategy, including both indirect services (planning and coordination) and direct services (counseling, health care, and social services), also assigns a special status to the providers of services. Again, Coser provides a vivid and accurate description: "Social workers, . . . administrators, and local volunteer workers seek out the poor in order to help them, yet, paradoxically, they are the very agents of their degradation. Subjective intentions and institutional consequences diverge here. The help rendered may be given from the purest and most benevolent of motives, yet the very fact of being helped degrades" (1963, p. 145). The problem is further compounded for the aged, the poor, or other recipients of services: "The professionals and [the client] . . . belong to two basically different worlds . . . and the asymmetry is not only of feelings and attitudes, it is also an asymmetry of power" (pp. 146–147). Because of their policy-defined unilateral dependency, the aged may in fact become more psychologically and socially dependent than they otherwise would. What is most significant is that the policies and programs established by the Older Americans Act encompass far more than their intended overt outcomes would indicate. These policies are critical, for they can reach inside the life experiences of the older person and severely limit his or her potential for self-sufficiency.

The creation of service bureaucracies also requires that a certain class of people be defined as in need, and this "definition must be broad enough so that the potential clientele is greater than the agency's capacity to provide the services" (Gordon and others, 1974, p. 5). Agency managers also seek control over definitions of problems, try to persuade clients that the services they provide are needed, and often limit information and accountability to the public by arguing that only providers are competent to evaluate their work. If evaluation is required, the focus is likely to be on processes, methods, and systems, not on outcomes. The development of trained specialties and licensing procedures that protect the work of professions is also likely.

Political consequences ensue. Perhaps most important is that use of the term *helping* obfuscates the political component of the roles being enacted, covering its repressive nature (Edelman, 1977). The use of terms such as *help* symbolically removes the political connotation of power that, in and of itself, might rally opposition instead of support. Rather than labeling an authority relationship as tyrannical, the professional defines the relationship as a helping relationship. Definition of the helping mode, the service, as a form of therapeutic assistance suggests that, if the necessary condition of submission to authority is met, the patient, the client, the aged person will benefit. The lay public comes to accept the professional's perspective for a variety of reasons, including its belief that experts can be trusted to handle problems, and this acceptance "is the politically crucial one, for it confers power upon professionals and spreads their norms to others" (Edelman, 1977, p. 67).

Crises and the Politics of Old Age

Social, economic, and political stakes are involved when social problems are represented as having reached a crisis stage. This view challenges conventional assumptions about the "objective" and nonpolitical origins of crises that come to national attention. My argument is not that there are conspiracies to create crises nor that crises result accidentally. Rather, crises are socially constructed as a consequence of social perception and definition; that is, a crisis comes to exist if it is perceived to exist. Conversely, a crisis does not exist if people do not act as though it exists. The definition of any given crisis is thus problematic.

Organized interests may seize upon opportunities to define as crises various problems (for which they claim to provide remedies) because of the significant economic and political resources that may be engendered by publicly acknowledged crises. This principle is demonstrated by an impressive catalogue of recent events, including the missile crisis, the environmental crisis, and the health care crisis. However, the role that organized interests play in defining a crisis is not always evident, as Edelman has made clear: "The long-term developments that make it possible for strategically located groups to precipitate a crisis, unintentionally or deliberately, are always complex and ambiguous. People who benefit from a crisis are usually able to explain it to themselves and to the mass public in terms that mask or minimize their own contributions and incentives, while highlighting outside threats and unexpected occurrences. The divergence between the symbolic import of crises and their material impact is basic to their popular acceptance" (1977, p. 46).

Past crises and the remembrance of them constitute an important impetus for future action; they often permit broad discretion by government and foster a public willingness to tolerate given actions to deal with the perceived crisis. Actions by government that would ordinarily be strongly resisted are often readily accepted in response to a defined crisis. The labeling of a problem as a crisis has many political uses (Edelman, 1964; 1971; 1977; Alford, 1976). The term *crisis* implies that the event or condition so described is different from others; that it is created by circumstances beyond the control of national leaders, who nevertheless are presumed to be coping with it in the best way possible; and that both action and sacrifice are required (Edelman, 1977, p. 44). In discussing the impacts of a crisis, Edelman argues, however, that "the burdens of almost all crises fall disproportionately on the poor, while the influential and the affluent often benefit from them" (1977, p. 44).

To define old age as a social problem of crisis proportions is politically useful because such a crisis may be portrayed as not the fault of prior social inaction or economic policy, but as the result of increased longevity, retirement, declining birth rates, and so forth. In addition to being amenable to characterization and explanation in ways which relieve politicians and bureaucrats of responsibility for its origins and career, the aging crisis label serves to advance the interests of those seeking expansion of government resources to deal with the crisis.

In addition, the aging crisis is easily characterized as requiring sacrifices. While appearing to be equally shared, such policy-delineated sacrifices are differentially borne—that is, the burdens of this crisis are not equally shared by rich and poor. This point is illustrated by the fact that policies for the aged do not seriously redress the disparities in income, status, housing, or employment. Thus, the designation process for labeling crises, in and of itself, is worthy of empirical investigation for understanding not only the policies that result but also their consequences for the aged, which in many instances may be at a very deep and personal level.

Comfort (1976b) describes the symbolic magnification of aging problems as one type of exploitation of the aged. Extremely negative portrayals of aging provide the basis for dramatizing old-age problems and for arguing that they constitute a crisis. Unfortunately, such portrayals are not without their negative effects on the aged themselves, as illustrated by the National Council on Aging study (1975) that was based on a nationwide Harris poll. The aged who were interviewed were the most negative of all age groups, describing older persons as passive, inert, functionally disabled, and sexless, although they tended to see themselves as exceptions to this characterization. Younger persons also viewed old age as a largely decremental and negative time of life. The crisis view of old age, then, can have the effect of deflating the self-esteem and denying the competency of aged individuals through service policies generating dependency while increasing their susceptibility to social control through regulation by service bureaucracies.

Contradictory Myths

In policies for the aged, there are two underlying but opposing perceptions or myths concerning "the problem"; these represent a basic ambivalance toward the causation of, and solution to, the problems that the government seeks to address. One conception defines the aged as responsible for their own plight and characterizes them (by inference) as immoral. In this view the aged are somehow culpable because they have not saved enough, not worked hard enough, or have lived too long. This conception calls for a minimal but official intervention of authorities and concerned professionals to protect society from the threat of dependency and unrest that the undeserving elderly may pose. Another conception sees the aged as victims of an exploitative economic and political system—victims, that is, of circumstances beyond their control. This conception calls for broad-scale substantive policies that would either alter their regrettable circumstances or "make up" (provide equity) for the hardship generated by society that the aged do not deserve but must endure.

The availability of such alternative explanations and their very consideration by public officials and professionals engender a continuing ambivalence and contradiction in public policy. While such contradictions are rooted in social inequality and reflect conflicting interests, they also provide a mechanism for resolving tensions. The coexistence of these diametrically opposed views has two consequences. First, it allows policies, whether successful or unsuccessful, to remain politically viable almost indefinitely. This occurs because, as citizens feel threatened and powerless to deal with complex problems, they welcome evidence of strong leadership, thus permitting "leaders to maintain power through a dramaturgy of coping, regardless of results" (Edelman, 1977, p. 147). Second, individuals can simultaneously know of large-scale conditions affecting their lives, yet individually blame themselves for their failures to successfully negotiate beyond those constraining conditions. For example, unemployed persons can hold the belief that they are personal failures yet simultaneously be aware of unemployment problems on a national or local scale but not relate these larger economic conditions to their personal or private troubles.

Contradictory interpretations of the cause, content, and solution to social problems create both ambivalence and psychological anxiety. These, in turn, create a need for reassurance, which political leaders willingly provide. The multiple realities and the recognition of alternative truths (each of which has some merit) provide the "continuation of broad public support for recurrent policies regardless of their empirical consequences. Ambivalence in the individual, ambiguity in political situations, and contradictory beliefs about problems and authority reinforce one another whenever governments deal with controversial issues" (Edelman, 1977, p. 142).

These acceptances of contradictory myths, explanations, and beliefs permit individuals to "play the role society demands while at the same time maintaining a measure of personal integrity by recognizing facts inconsistent with the role . . . [In this way] people survive by occupying coexisting 'realities' that only rarely disturb each other" (Edelman, 1977, p. 151).

Specifically, the objectives of the Older Americans Act include enabling the aged to live independently with adequate income, giving them opportunities for leisure, employment, and decent housing, and making it possible for them to maximize their health and develop their potential. These objectives, which imply the "right" of the aged to enjoy certain benefits and standards in society, stand in stark opposition to what the Older Americans Act actually provides the aged. Thus, this legislation actually contains a pair of opposing myths and definitions about the elderly. If the aged are cast as deserving because they are caught in a situation beyond their control, the service strategies embodied in the act tend to define the aged as passive dependents who must be "helped." An explicit definition of the aged as responsible for their own plight (and therefore somehow immoral) is absent, but the asymmetrical power relationships involved in the giving and receiving of services (as opposed to an adequate income that would permit the aged to negotiate society in a more equal position) are scarcely based upon a conception of the aged as dignified individuals with incontrovertible rights in society.

Thus, political pronouncements such as the Older Americans Act answer the underlying need of the public to understand a complex world and to be reassured that their leaders are responding to the very problems that have been socially created and defined, in large part by the leaders themselves.

The symbolic aspects of the goals of the Older Americans Act reassure the public that somehow the aged are being cared for, while policy is simultaneously constructed so that its material impact will not disrupt the ongoing functioning or power arrangements within society. The intentionally ambiguous language of the Older Americans Act prevents both a clear understanding of the problem and the testing of alternatives. But because the problem appears to have been defined and solutions undertaken, a constriction of policy choice results. Once set in motion, policy choices are weighted in the direction of incremental change and will be largely limited to efforts at fine tuning and the adjustment of existing strategies.

If a national policy that will improve life for the aged is ever to be developed it will have to resolve the basic ambiguities and confusions of the Older Americans Act and give reality to the hopes that the Act symbolizes. Whatever the failures of the Older Americans Act, however, the programs and policies that it mandates require a closer scrutiny than we have yet given them.

III

Sociopolitical Influences
on the Development of
the Older Americans Act

═══════◦▭◦════════◦▭◦═══════

*The goal of the Older Americans Act . . . is to enable older people
to live in their own homes as independently as possible. The strategy that
was conceived to reach that goal is coordination. . . It is as if we said that
it is in the public interest to provide each citizen with the opportunity for
full employment . . . and then announced that . . . to reach that goal we
were going to coordinate training programs* [Brinnon, 1975, p. 4].

The Older Americans Act was one of several major federal initiatives in the 1960s designed specifically to benefit the elderly. Many
of the other programs enacted as part of President Johnson's Great
Society legislation purportedly were to benefit the elderly, since
it is a fact that a great many of the aged are poor. The Older
Americans Act initially was a reflection of the brief period of intense legislative activity from 1963 to 1966 that broke new ground
in federal policies related to civil rights, health, education, environmental quality, consumer protection, model cities, and other

Note: Many ideas in this chapter are drawn from Estes, Armour,
and Noble (1977); and from Armour, Estes, and Noble (1978).

31

areas of domestic policy. This period of activism and change was in sharp contrast to the tradition of incrementalism in federal policy. Only in two other periods in the twentieth century (the first terms of Woodrow Wilson's and of Franklin D. Roosevelt's presidencies) was there anything like it in American politics.

The federal government's activist role in social policy resulted in legislation across a broad front, as well as in rapidly increasing expenditures on old age income transfer programs—Old Age Survivors Insurance and Medicare, for example. Not only were existing programs modified and expanded, but the federal government also enacted and attempted to implement new social programs on a massive scale. The Community Mental Health Centers, Comprehensive Health Planning, Medicare, Medicaid, Economic Opportunity, Civil Rights, Elementary and Secondary Education, and Model Cities acts testify to the social welfare policy commitment that emerged in the 1960s.

Many of these programs defined new political and administrative jurisdictions, at times by creating paragovernments (policy-making bodies outside of local government), even as they emphasized participatory decision making. The health care and social service programs advocated technical planning tempered by the pragmatism of local politics, so that the new services would be better coordinated with related service programs (Marris and Rein, 1967). Whether designed to enfranchise new participants (such as consumers, elders, or poor people) through formal political institutions and elected officials or through measures that involved consumers, these programs evoked an ethos of public accountability.

The goals were to be achieved through a variety of funding mechanisms: categorical grants, block grants, formula grants, social insurance, and even vouchers. Some programs required an income test for eligibility; others did not. A common theme in many of the programs was increased community involvement in solving socioeconomic problems, while mobilizing local resources for new and expanded social services. National policy sought to expand and alter qualitatively the traditional role of local government and community institutions.

As mentioned earlier, the Older Americans Act and Medicare were both designed specifically to deal with problems of the aged, but the strategies of the two programs differed dramatically:

Medicare was to pay for hospital and physician services for the elderly, while the Older Americans Act had more global objectives. Like many of the Great Society programs, the latter's goals far exceeded its legislative authority and subsequent appropriations. Title I of the 1965 Older Americans Act, for example, stated ten broad objectives for the elderly:

1. An adequate income in retirement,
2. The best possible physical and mental health,
3. Suitable housing,
4. Full restorative services for those who need institutional care,
5. Employment without age discrimination,
6. Retirement in health, honor, and dignity,
7. Participation in civic, cultural, and recreational activities,
8. Efficient community services, which provide social assistance in a coordinated manner and which are readily available when needed,
9. Immediate benefit from research,
10. Free exercise of individual initiative in planning and managing one's own life.

The Older Americans Act established a small operating agency, the Administration on Aging, which created three operating programs: grants to states for community service projects (Title III), research and demonstration projects (Title IV), and training programs (Title V). Title III provided funds to create an agency on aging in each state to plan, coordinate, and develop services. In most states these agencies became small grant-making units rather than focal points for advocacy or development of services. Title IV stipulated that grants and contracts be made to public and private nonprofit organizations to study the status of older people and to demonstrate approaches for improving conditions and bettering the coordination of community services. Title V specified that grants and contracts be awarded to public and private nonprofit agencies and organizations for training and developing curriculums designed to assist persons employed in programs related to the act.

Although both the Economic Opportunity Act and the Older Americans Act were important elements in President Johnson's

Great Society program and contained some of the same basic strategies, there were fundamental differences in their approaches. One important difference was the political visibility given the Office of Economic Opportunity (OEO). The OEO was set up in the White House itself, and the director reported to the president. The Administration on Aging, in contrast, was contained within the Social and Rehabilitation Services (SRS) in the Department of Health, Education, and Welfare (HEW); and the commissioner reported to the SRS administrator, who in turn reported to the HEW secretary.

The fate of the Economic Opportunity Act of 1964 would profoundly affect that of the later phases of the Older Americans Act. The Economic Opportunity Act attempted to reform and reorient major social institutions—for example, education, social welfare services, health care, and manpower training—to provide equity in the allocation of resources, access to service, and institutional responsiveness (Levitan, 1969). In its early years, mandates were broad and goals were ill defined. Goals included the identification, coordination, and consolidation of local resources, including social services, into a comprehensive system responsive to the poor.

One strategy adopted by the OEO was developing paragovernments, which enfranchised previously underrepresented citizen groups by creating consumer boards and advisory councils. It was hoped that the OEO, using the participatory paradigm, could mount a direct attack on the indifferent bureaucratic structures of public programs for the poor. A second strategy was employing technical planning expertise to identify needs, acquire resources, and provide legitimacy to new paragovernmental citizen boards. However, implementing rational, comprehensive planning had to be deemphasized in the face of urgent local demands for immediate, observable results in the form of jobs, services, and programs.

Numerous problems plagued OEO programs. OEO's goal of consumer participation was often in direct conflict with the goal of basing decision making on planning criteria. A primary problem was that rational planning required cooperation from the community, specifically of service and political organizations over which OEO planners had no authority, and such cooperation was not obtained. The right of the community action programs to make decisions concerning existing services, a right which by-passed other formal procedures, was also controversial and difficult to implement. Lacking legitimacy to enforce comprehensive rational planning as a basis for changing local decisions, the original community action programs turned to "politicking" as the only strategy for affecting or directing local services.

Barriers to reforms on the local level were strong enough to significantly influence the proverty program's future. As a consequence of heightened expectations and demands, intensified politics, severe disappointments, and the change of administrations in Washington, the Economic Opportunity Act has been radically altered, and many community action programs now resemble large, multipurpose service agencies, rather than the planning and advocacy organizations originally envisioned. The OEO was abolished during the Nixon administration; its remaining functions were transferred to the Community Services Administration in the Department of Health, Education, and Welfare. This swing of the pendulum from activism to incrementalism, from direct federal involvement to decentralization and local control, was to be reflected in many other policies and programs—including the Older Americans Act.

Amendments in 1969 to the Older Americans Act gave new authority under Title III for the commissioner on aging to fund model projects and assigned state units on aging specific responsibility for planning, coordinating, and evaluating services within their states. It also added a new Title VI to establish volunteer programs to aid the elderly. In 1972, a new Title VII established nutrition programs for the elderly.

By 1973 the time had arrived for a more basic reconsideration of the Older Americans Act, particularly the Grants to States for Community Service Projects under Title III. The forerunners of this reconsideration were the planning and decentralization policies of the Economic Opportunity Act of 1964 and the State and Local Fiscal Assistance Act of 1972 (general revenue sharing). Both of these acts sought—if in vastly different ways—to integrate technical planning with administrative and political decentralization. The 1973 amendments to the Older Americans Act created area agencies on aging as decentralized bodies with the broad mandates of planning, coordinating, and pooling local resources as well as of funding a small number of gap-filling services. These were just the kinds of goals not achieved by the community action program of OEO. The decentralization of decision making and the local discretion provided in setting priorities under an ambitious but also amibiguous Older Americans Act mandate were similar to the authority granted state and local governments under the State and Local Fiscal Assistance Act of 1972.

The most controversial aspect of the OEO strategy—citizen policy boards—was dropped entirely in the Older Americans Act. Instead, consumer participation was mandated in the form of advisory councils, first in 1965 to state units on aging and then to nutrition projects in 1972. In 1973 mandates for advisory assistance from elders were adopted at the federal and area levels. Although they are required to review and comment on state and area plans, any other involvement of advisory groups in the work of state units, nutrition, or area agencies is a matter of agency discretion. Federal regulations concerning these advisory bodies are interpreted by the Administration on Aging as prohibiting their assumption of policy-making roles (Estes, 1975b).

Although the Economic Opportunity Act of 1964 did not achieve many of its early goals, it did have a major impact on public policy and the public's perception of the poverty problem. It also served as a catalyst to efforts to legislate a national policy on aging. This and other New Frontier–Great Society social welfare policies served: (1) to legitimate a policy for a clientele group based on advanced age, just as the OEO program and its predecessor, Mobilization for Youth, had been aimed primarily at the young; (2) to dramatize socioeconomic deprivation in America; (3) to define the federal government's role in providing opportunities for the impoverished to improve their lot; (4) to institutionalize a reform model based on the assumed benefits of the rational planning and coordination of social services; and (5) to decentralize responsibility for making the program work. The Older Americans Act policy of universal eligibility without regard to differential need was a consequence primarily of OEO's claim to already serve the poor. To avoid a duplicative approach to the aged, the Older Americans Act addressed not just the poor, but all the aged (Estes and Gerard, 1978a).

The 1970s and the Older Americans Act

The centerpiece of the Nixon administration's strategy was to limit federal involvement in domestic social programs and to decentralize the programs to provide for local control though the State and Local Fiscal Assistance Act of 1972, commonly known as the general revenue sharing act. The overt premise of this act was that local governments know best how to meet local needs. Its intended effect was neither the enfranchisement of new groups nor the development of new planning and decision-making bodies controlled by such groups. Rather, it was meant to strengthen state and local governments by direct transfers of revenues from the federal government and the elimination of the strings usually attached to federal grants. This was a dramatic departure from the policies of the 1960s, with their emphasis on categorical grants that left relatively little leeway for pragmatic decisions by state and local governments.

The larger framework for understanding the policy heritage of the Older Americans Act can be found in the American federal system itself, together with recent American policy configurations that attempt to augment state and local autonomy. The reimposition of a federalist strategy in the 1970s was an effort to resolve, first of all, the problem of an impending national-level economic crisis coincidental with increased pressures from state and local governments, whose tax revenues were leveling off, for more federal funding. Secondly, there was the inability of the federal government to meet the increasing service demands of groups enfranchised and conscious of their rights as a consequence of social programs of the 1960s. New federalism provided President Nixon with a mechanism for channeling the participatory demands of the 1960s into a local control strategy and for diffusing the potential concentration of power among newly enfranchised but discontented groups.

The tensions and dilemmas inherent in the design and implementation of the Older Americans Act itself seem to emanate from three somewhat contradictory policy heritages: (1) the categorical grant-in-aid to states (an approach embodied in the Older

Americans Act of 1965, as well as in the 1967 and 1969 amendments and the Title VII nutrition program enacted in 1972); (2) efforts to achieve institutional change through the Poverty and Model Cities Programs, which gradually incorporated the rationalizing forces of planning in order to moderate the demands arising from citizen participation; and (3) the principle of decentralization embodied in the new federalism, of which general and special revenue sharing are primary examples.

The 1973 Comprehensive Service Amendments to the Older Americans Act were powerfully affected by President Nixon's new federalism strategy of the 1970s. This influence is apparent in the emphasis given to local decision making through the creation of area agencies on aging under the administration of state units on aging, as well as in the discretion for block-grant funding that area agencies received in these 1973 amendments. The definitions in the service amendments of the relationships between state and local agencies on aging provide a rudimentary articulation of the means for implementing a decentralized national social program for the elderly. The wide variability permitted in administrative and organizational structures is illustrative of the new federalism strategy. State units on aging vary from cabinet-level departments in some states to separate commissions or divisions within the governor's office in others, but most states created subunits of larger health and welfare agencies. The state units have direct responsibility for administering and monitoring their contracts with the area agencies, including development of allocation formulas. They also have responsibility for the development of statewide aging services plans for Title III and for nutrition programs within their states. The state agencies had responsibility for the direct administration of nutrition services and senior centers until the Comprehensive Older Americans Act Amendments of 1978 consolidated Titles III (area planning and social services), V (senior centers), and VII (nutrition), granting more decision-making authority to area agencies. But state units continue to administer the statewide area agency programs and to assess and monitor the activities of area agencies. In addition, they still coordinate and pool resources for existing state-level programs. Given the emphasis on area agencies and local programs, however, state units have little time for leadership activities beyond administrative responsibilities for the area agencies.

The Older Americans Act allows considerable autonomy in the application of federal guidelines in designating planning and service area boundaries, defining target populations, and operationalizing standards. The national program aims at developing services through decentralized decision making and the setting of funding priorities. This assures variability in the implementation process, which is beneficial to the extent that it enables localities to deal with their unique problems unhampered by federal regulations. Lack of federal control, however, also frees agencies from certain requirements—for example, addressing the needs of the more disadvantaged aged. As determined by the planning process, priorities may or may not be reflected in the grants for services— these priorities being more likely determined by local politics and negotiation than by rational planning (Estes, 1975b). In addition, the limited funding available for direct services under Title III provides little incentive for local funding of high-cost direct services, such as daycare programs, which do not yield the visible return in large numbers of claimed units of service such as information and referral services or transportation services do.

Area agencies were given a broad mandate to develop area service plans, to expand services by pooling resources, to coordinate existing services, and, where necessary, to fund gap-filling services for the aged. Area agencies are directly responsible to the unit of state government through which their funds are channeled, and many are also responsible to units of local government. While most area agencies are public agencies, many are private, nonprofit agencies with no direct tie to local government. Out of a recent sample of 229 responding public area agencies, 45 percent were located in regional planning commissions or economic development districts, and 38.4 percent were located under the auspices of county governments. Of the 148 private, nonprofit area agencies, 56.1 percent were independent agencies, while less than 17 percent were under the auspices of a regional planning commission (U.S. House, 1978e). In half a dozen rural states the state unit on aging is also the area agency on aging, and many area agencies include several counties within their jurisdiction.

Area planning and social services agencies also vary in the types of services they fund. In 1973 the Administration on Aging emphasized the access services of escort, outreach, transportation, and information and referral. In that same year Congress set minimum Title III funding requirements for four priority services: legal aid, home repair, in-home services, and transportation. Congressional imposition of national priority services continued to be an issue during the 1978 Older Americans Act reauthorization debate, since it was argued that these national priorities infringed on the discretion of area agencies to plan and develop services designed to meet the special needs within a specific area. Nevertheless, priority emphasis for access services, health and in-home services, and legal assistance was part of the 1978 amendment language.

The policy goals of area planning are to secure and maintain maximum independence in the community for older persons and to prevent their institutionalization. The intervention strategy, or program, embodied in Title III has two foci. The primary intervention focus is an institutional change strategy aimed at improving and expanding the existing service delivery system through the "indirect" services of planning, coordination, and pooling. The second focus is the direct delivery of services through small grants at the area agency level; this strategy is a primary intervention designed to improve the access of individuals to services that affect their daily functioning. For example, meals-on-wheels programs forestall physical deterioration by delivering balanced meals to elders unable to take care of their own nutritional needs. The question that must be raised about both of these strategies is, Can they succeed? Has either one identified the causal variables that are likely to produce the maximum desired change in the life of the aged? In both cases the ultimate policy goal is to reduce inappropriate institutionalization and maximize the independence of the aged.

At the heart of the institutional change strategy is a planning component that presents problems of its own. The underlying assumptions of this strategy are that rationality can be approximated and that there is a system that planners need to coordinate. Planning is a modest intervention strategy, for it treats problems by modifying noneconomic factors in the environment and looks upon the manipulation of architectural and other environmental features as primary interventions. Existing power relationships are taken as given and the "public or collective good" is assumed to be achievable through the promotion of planning. This view of the world overemphasizes the nonsocial and noneconomic aspects of situations.

Coordination, the second element of the institutional change strategy, encompasses activities undertaken by state and area agencies to encourage communication among existing service providers, integration of services, and other joint efforts that improve access to the use of services. Emphasis has been on communication and exchange of information, since state units and area agencies have no authority to compel cooperation or coordination on the part of independent agencies.

Pooling has caused the most conceptual confusion of all mandated responsibilities under the institutional change strategy. Generally, pooling refers to those activities or efforts undertaken by area agencies and state units to stimulate the allocation of state or local money to expand services for the aged. Originally referred to in federal guidelines as "pooling and tapping" resources, pooling includes development of special grants and proposals and advocating for fair-share allocations for aging services in various budgets—for example, Title XX (Social Security Act) social services, revenue sharing, and community development block grants.

No clear indication of the relative weight to be given institutional change or direct services intervention strategies is evident in the Title III guidelines. Nevertheless, the institutional change strategy has assumed prominence in the national debate.

At the local level, however, the preference for the allocation of Title III funds to direct services has been voiced by elderly citizens as well as by local administrators and politicians. Faced with increasing demands for services and limited resources, locally elected officials are less inclined to consider reorganization and rationalization of service delivery through planning and coordination as priorities. Designed originally as a seed-grant program to encourage local spending for aging services, Title III is, in fact, becoming the major (although small) source of support for such services, particularly as limits are being set at the national, state, and local levels for service expenditures. The passage of California's Jarvis-Gann Tax Initiative in 1978 and similar efforts in other states to reduce the tax revenues available to local government will create even more pressure for area agencies on aging to use their meager funds for direct services. Furthermore, Title III dollars so spent produce visible outputs—units of service and number of elders served. The direct services strategy with its immediate and tangible impact makes localities appear to be "doing something." In contrast, the effects of the institutional change strategy are less easily substantiated, and it has the added disadvantage of requiring a longer time span before results can be seen.

Serious doubt has been raised as to whether either of these strategies, but especially the planning and coordination (institutional change) strategy, is of potential benefit to America's elders. Many problems of the aged do not result from local failures in planning, coordination, and service integration, as the Title III institutional change strategy assumes. The problem is far more complex and must be addressed on the federal as well as the state and local levels. Given the federal limitations on funds for Social Security, Supplementary Security Income, Title XX social services, and Medicare, a small, fragmented grant program such as Title III will not have much effect in meeting the needs of the aged. It can have no effect on federal policies related to the employment of the aged, their medical care, or the level of their Social Security benefits. Some also criticize the direct service strategy of Title III for its ad hoc proliferation of aging services and for supporting the development of parallel and competing aging service systems. This strategy, so the argument goes, ignores the critical tasks of increasing access to, and improving the responsiveness of, existing service systems for the aged, while also contributing to services fragmentation.

Since the 1973 Comprehensive Services Amendments were enacted, questions concerning the concept and performance of the Title III institutional change strategy have been raised in numerous hearings, especially by the House Select Committee on Aging and the Senate Special Committee on Aging (Estes and Gerard, 1978a). In 1975 Congressman John Brademas asked the most specific and extensive questions about the effectiveness of the institutional change strategy and about the causal theories underlying the area planning and social services program (U.S. House, 1975):

1. What are the relative merits of direct services versus planning, coordination, and pooling functions?
2. Is the strategy working? Is there any evidence with regard to this? What evaluation studies of area agency on aging program performance have been undertaken? What is the evidence of area agency pooling performance of general revenue sharing funds?
3. How feasible is it for communities to pick up the tab after expiration of the three-year limit on social services funding under Title III?
4. Who benefits? What are the statistics on the socioeconomic status of older persons benefiting? Are low-income elderly actually receiving benefits?
5. Are we satisfied with the current mix of funds allocated to services and to administration? Why are coordination and pooling defined by the Administration on Aging as services instead of administrative costs?

The responses to this extensive inquiry ranged from emphasizing that the program strategy was too new in 1975 to yield any hard evidence to verbal reassurance from the national associations of state and area agencies concerning the soundness of the approach. When asked about the efficacy of the Older Americans Act planning and coordination strategy, given the history of such relatively unsuccessful programs as Comprehensive Health Planning and Model Cities, Arthur Flemming, U.S. commissioner on aging, reassured Congressman Brademas: "The Area Planning and Social Services program is distinguishable in many respects from these programs. We took into account many of their experiences when we developed the policies and guidelines for the Title III Programs. There is no conclusive evidence relative to the operations of the area agencies on aging on which basis we could make comparisons with the other program" (U.S. House, 1975, p. 113).

Despite this kind of official optimism, serious doubts remain about the conceptualization and design of the area planning and social services strategy. There may be tenuous links between the direct service and institutional change strategies of Title III and the policy goals of assuring independence and preventing institutionalization of the aged, but these links are not apparent.

1978 Reauthorization

In the limited debate about the 1978 reauthorization of the Older Americans Act, little consideration was given to basic reform. What little deliberation there was primarily reinforced the existing power relationships among the interest groups that have come to some accommodation since passage of the 1973 Comprehensive Services Amendments. The agencies legislatively defined as appropriate caretakers of the aged each put forth demands for a share of the taken-for-granted Older Americans Act resources. The predominant characteristics of the debate were minor conflicts over those adjustments seen as necessary by various parties to the aging network—a network comprised not of the aged but of the agencies. Submerged but still persistent are the problems of accountability under the Older Americans Act—the vagueness and ambiguity of objectives, the difficulty of evaluation given the multiple broad goals of the act, and the conflicting causal theories and strategies. One can add to this the shared cynicism of elders, network members, policy makers, and the public.

The general themes in the Older Americans Act reauthorization testimony provide continuing basic support for policies enunciated in the 1973 amendments, with a recurrent emphasis on the presumed benefits of decentralization and the merits of the planning and coordination services strategies. As evidenced by testimony in favor of even more area agency discretion through block-grant funding, little attention was accorded to national objectives, national standards, or to the targeting of resources to subpopulations of the aged in greatest need. There was an apparent lack of concern for coherent policies and national strategies. Instead, short-term, routine problem-solving approaches dominated the reauthorization debate, undoubtedly because these are the central and direct concerns of state and area agencies—now among the major organized interests influencing policy on the aging. These agencies, together with the organized providers, professionals, service contractors, and national membership organizations, were the dominant actors in the debates. Analysis of reauthorization testimony reveals a limited vision of the possible and one heavily influenced by the assumption that the act's area planning and coordination strategy, nutrition programs, senior centers, and limited employment programs are both beneficial and appropriate approaches to the problems of the aged (Estes and Gerard, 1978b).

The three key concepts of the Older Americans Act incorporated into programs and policies of the 1960s and into the new federalism strategy of the early 1970s continue in the 1978 Older Americans Act Amendments: (1) a decentralized approach to federal-state-local relations; (2) a clientele approach with universal eligibility (that is, all elderly are eligible for services, and there is no targeting of resources for the most disadvantaged); and (3) the adoption of a planning and coordination services strategy.

Hearings on the 1978 reauthorization before the House Select Committee on Aging in 1977 witnessed overwhelming support for the current design of the Title III strategy; however, the committee did not probe for evidence of the effectiveness of this approach or for any opinions other than those presented by the area agencies themselves. Thus, while questions about the effectiveness of the planning and coordinating strategy have been raised (U.S. Senate, 1978b; Benedict, 1978; U.S. House, 1975), the Title III strategy was neither seriously challenged nor significantly altered in the 1978 amendments; in fact, there was overwhelming support for maintaining the current approach despite a paucity of data concerning its efficacy.

The main thrust of the deliberations on the Comprehensive Older Americans Act Amendments of 1978 was concerned with efficiency and effectiveness, hinging on issues of coordination and decentralization. To address the ongoing question of the Administration on Aging's power and authority to fulfill its mandate to coordinate programs and to be at the federal level a focal point on aging, the 1978 amendments included for the first time a provision requiring that programs within the Administration on Aging be coordinated with other major federal programs in health, housing, labor, transportation, and social services. Efforts to redress the problems of fragmentation and conflict that developed at the local level within the aging network itself are evidenced by the consolidation of Titles III (area planning and social services), V (multipurpose senior centers), and VII (nutrition services), as well as by language that encourages area agencies to designate, wherever feasible, a focal point agency for the delivery of comprehensive coordinated services within the community. These changes were intended to lessen paperwork burdens, streamline the planning process, and improve coordination of services. Consequently, a good deal more discretionary authority was granted to the area agencies. Another issue under the rubric of coordination and planning was whether area agencies should engage in a more direct service strategy. The rationale presented during the 1975 and 1978 reauthorization hearings, one which continues to prevail, is that the provision of direct services by area agencies would make them competitive with existing service providers and would hamper their work as coordinators.

The issue of decentralization continued to be a salient one. Congress reexamined the need to balance national objectives with flexibility and discretion at the local level. The four national service priorities mandated in 1975 were widely challenged, and many reaffirmed the viability of the basic premise of the new federalism—"those in charge of local programs are in the best position to identify local problems and can thus apply federal funds where they are needed most" (*Congressional Record,* 1978, p. S11592). Many national aging organizations argued that mandated national priorities contradicted the intent of Title III, which allows area and state agencies to develop plans according to the needs of the community. Likewise, a U.S. General Accounting Office report (1978) emphasized the ineffectiveness of national priority areas, concluding that they had a negative effect by causing additional financial and administrative problems in program reporting.

Robert Binstock's widely discussed proposal was essentially a block-grant program in which area agencies would have the discretion to determine concentrated program priority areas in accordance with their own perceptions of the most pressing local concerns related to the needs of older persons. The justification for this was that it "might enable services to the aging to develop as a concentrated response to priority crises experienced by older persons . . . rather than as minimum, token coverage of a large range of possibilities identified by professionals" (Binstock, in U.S. Senate, 1978a, p. 6). Others, such as the National Association of Counties, argued vigorously for a pass-through of funds from the federal to the local level in block-grant funding that would by-pass both state and area agencies, while state and area agencies, along with many service providers, argued jointly that area agencies must continue.

A recent study conducted by the Administration on Aging, however, indicated that "services continue to be widely dispersed and unfocused at the local level, [a situation] which often renders scarce resources diffused and ineffective at meeting the needs of older Americans" (*Congressional Record*, 1978, p. S11561). Thus, despite vigorous arguments to the contrary, Congress upheld the inclusion of priority services in the interest of more efficient and effective use of scarce resources. The 1978 amendments resulted in a compromise solution requiring that at least 50 percent of Title III funds be expended for access services, transportation, outreach, information and referral, and in-home and legal services. At the same time, it gave the local level the discretion to determine which proportion of the 50 percent is to be targeted to each of these services.

Another area in which state and local discretion remained intact was the targeting of resources to elderly persons who were economically disadvantaged or members of minorities. The 1978 amendments reiterate support for a clientele approach premised on universal eligibility for all older Americans and effectively eliminated proposals that would have targeted resources to the poor and minorities, either through a change in the allotment formula or the mandated targeting of services at the local level. The 1978 amendments suggest only that preference be given to those in greatest economic or social need. The notion advanced was that social and economic needs are commensurate, that is, that social needs are just as important as economic needs; therefore, it is left to the discretion of area agencies to determine which needs of the elderly have priority in their local communities (U.S. House, 1978h).

While the act continues to deemphasize any class differences among older Americans, the 1978 reauthorization hearings gave attention to geographic differences between the rural and urban elderly, as well as to vulnerable groups of elderly requiring long-term health care. In contrast, economic impoverishment received little attention.

The 1978 amendments include a provision to retain the existing state formula but add a requirement that each state reserve from its allotment an additional 5 percent above the amount it is currently spending on services to rural areas; in addition, model projects and research studies are to emphasize the special needs of the rural elderly. A new authority was created, permitting the commissioner on aging to fund model projects "to demonstrate innovative approaches to comprehensive and coordinated long-term care delivery" (Congressional Record, 1978, p. S11538). The scope of long-term care ranges from adult daycare to supported living in public nonprofit housing and family respite services. Key provisions in the model-projects proposal include the need to "provide for identification and assessment of long-term care needs of individual elderly persons, referral of such persons to the appropriate services, follow-up and evaluation of the continued appropriateness of such services" (Congressional Record, 1978, p. S11538). But funds cannot be used to pay for direct services reimbursable under Title XVIII, Title XIX, or Title XX of the Social Security Act. Hence, if these restrictions are rigorously imposed, many of the long-term care projects funded under this authority would provide information and referral services rather than the needed long-term and direct care services.

Long-term care demonstrations that focus expenditure on specific policy goals have the effect of limiting eligibility. It would be possible to limit costs by targeting services to those elders who are most frail or vulnerable to institutionalization, instead of providing a little bit of aid for all older persons. But such a major reorientation of policy would be feasible only if national priorities were altered and financial support increased substantially. This would be consistent with Commissioner Benedict's (1978) call for changes in the funding mechanism for the area planning and social services programs. In place of the current categorical grant programs operated by the area agencies, he initially proposed a national system of unified reimbursement to the states that would cover all aging services, including intermediate and skilled nursing care. The regulatory and planning requirements of the strategy could be streamlined and simplified and lead to increased decentralization. However, the mandate to assess the long-term care needs of individual aged persons raises further questions: Will this program create a new group of bureaucratic certifiers who will control access of the elderly to services; to what extent will this demonstration authority limit rather than expand the access to community-based long-term care services; and to what extent will it stigmatize the elderly as frail or disabled?

Finally, one is led to ask, why have policy makers and political leaders fostered the organizational development and bureaucratic expansion of multiple aging networks under the Older Americans Act when this approach costs so much and raises so many questions? The answers lie, first, in the social construction of reality: The aged are seen as constituting a social problem that has reached a crisis. In the face of such a reality Congress and the executive branch feel the need to do something. Regardless of the efficacy of the national policy contained in the Older Americans Act, politicians can earnestly claim that they have created policies and appropriated funds, thereby giving needed attention to the problems and demands of the aged. Second, there is a large contingent of organized interest groups, many of which are part of the aging network created by the Older Americans Act and its amendments, that have limited their support to incremental changes in the 1978 reauthorization effort. Third, the Older Americans Act, as a largely symbolic response, fulfills both a co-optative social control function for the middle class and a disciplinary social control function for those of the aged who are poor.

The unquestioning acceptance of the area agency approach during the 1978 reauthorization debate reflects the continuing dominance of a strategy that minimizes activities that might create conflict among providers, state and community leaders, and other interest groups, and engenders short- rather than long-range goals. The approach is one that is likely to create only "a little bit of

change around the edges" (Lowi, 1971, p. xv). As such, it is politically appealing because there is "little cause for the formation of
clear politicial oppositions" (p. xv).

A Decade in Retrospect

Policies are implemented when authorized programs are
funded. The significant changes that the Older Americans Act has
undergone since its enactment in 1965 have been reflected in appropriations. Total appropriations have grown from the tiny sum
of $7.5 million in fiscal year 1966 to slightly more than $699 million
in fiscal year 1978, including the funds appropriated to the Department of Labor for the Senior Community Service Employment
Program. In the first three years, funding was available for state
agencies, community projects, research, training, and demonstration. Amendments in 1969 added model projects to Title III and
assigned state units on aging specific authority for planning, coordinating, and evaluating services for the aged within their states.
It also added Title VI, national older Americans volunteer programs. Important developments occurred in 1972 with the addition of the nutrition programs and in 1973 with the Comprehensive Services Amendments to Title III that created area agencies
on aging. In fiscal year 1973, total funding rose to $257 million,
from $101 million in fiscal year 1972 and $38 million in fiscal year
1971 (see Table 1).

Appropriations for volunteer and employment programs
are somewhat difficult to track during this period because the President's reorganization plan No. 1 of 1971 transferred the Foster
Grandparents and Senior Volunteer programs to the ACTION
agency, a newly formed citizens' service corps, and in 1973 the
Title VI of the Older Americans Act was repealed by the Domestic
Volunteer Service Act. Similarly, the Senior Community Service
Employment Program is authorized by the Other Americans Act
but is administered by the Department of Labor.

While Older Americans Act appropriations have grown dramatically since 1965 relative to standards of budget incrementalism, the absolute size of appropriations relative to the needs of the
aged remains woefully inadequate. The funding and appropria-

**Table 1. Older Americans Act Appropriation:
Fiscal Year 1975–Fiscal Year 1978**

Program	Appropriation (millions of dollars)			
	1975	*1976*	*1977*	*1978*
Title II				
National Clearinghouse				2
Federal Council on Aging				0.45
Title III				
Area Planning and Social Services	82	93	122	153
Model Projects	28	13.8	17	19
State Agency Operations	15	17	14.7	15
Title IV				
Training	8	10	14.2	17.0
Research	7	8	8.5	8.5
Multidisciplinary Centers of Gerontology		1	3.8	3.8
Title V				
Multipurpose Senior Centers			20	40.0
Title VII				
Nutrition	125	125	202	250
Title IX				
Community Service Employment	336.4[a]	55.9	90.6	190.4
Volunteer programs, administered by ACTION				
Retired Senior Volunteer Program	15.98		19	20.1
Foster Grandparents	28.28		34	34.9
Senior Companions	2.56		3.8	7.0

[a] 26.4 Operation Mainstream

tions history of the Older Americans Act illustrates the persistent struggle among the executive branch, Congress, and interest groups over a multitude of issues related to federal policies affecting the aged. In the absence of a coherent national policy on aging, such struggles are likely to continue as a large number of interest groups compete for scarce resources.

The total amount of funds to be appropriated remains a contested issue. Four main arguments have been advanced against increasing appropriations further: (1) the federal government cannot meet all the needs of the elderly population without going broke in deficit spending (it has done something, and that will have to be enough); (2) the planning, coordination, and gap-filling (Title III) funds are seed monies to enable state and area agencies to act as catalysts for needed programs with short-term, limited grants and as gatherers of (presumably) available state and local resources; (3) the Older Americans Act strategy of planning, coordination, and advocacy cannot meet the real needs of older people—health, income, and housing—and appropriations should be seen as merely symbolic gestures; and (4) the allocation of more federal resources for the elderly will create or contribute to intergenerational conflict.

Arguments that the government cannot meet all of the needs of the elderly without going broke were presented during the 1978 Older Americans Act reauthorization debate. Senator Harry Byrd pointed out that one of the proposed bills, S.2850, would authorize more than $1.2 billion for fiscal year 1979, adding to deficit spending, which is a major cause of inflation and thus contributes to the economic hardship of senior citizens (the proposed authorization increase would have been 47 percent). Assuming a yearly inflation rate from 1978 to 1979 of 8 percent, Senator Byrd argued that "this legislation is proposing an increase more than 5 times the inflation rate" (*Congressional Record*, 1978, p. S11592).

The thrust of the Title III seed-money concept was defined by a Nixon administration spokesman as follows: "Basically we think the federal money ought to be used to stimulate new activity, which is then picked up by state and local governments out of other revenues, and the federal government should then use its funds to stimulate still new ones . . . if instead we get in the business of continually supporting the same agencies and the same organizations and the same senators, . . . we will not reach the universal needs that we were talking about before" (Kurzman in U.S. House, 1973, p. 79).

The argument that area agencies on aging are catalysts to

stimulate the development of local resources assumes those resources are available or that providers who have been funded by
these agencies will continue to deliver their services after agency
funding stops. Such assumptions, of course, raise the question
whether there are sufficient available state or local resources to
pick up the tab. A quick review of testimony from the intergovernmental lobby, which is composed of mayors, governors, and local officials, would indicate that the answer is no. In fact, more and
more state and local officials are pressing the federal government
to assume more—not less—of the cost for health and social services
precisely because their resources are dwindling and a taxpayers'
revolt seems to be brewing, while the demands for services have
not dimished. Although there is reason to doubt the viability of
policies that reduce federal funding in order to "draw out" local
resources in view of the acknowledged fiscal strain on state and
local governments, Health, Education, and Welfare Secretary
Joseph Califano (in U.S. Senate, 1978b) ascribes some measure of
success to the efforts of service-coordinating state units and area
agencies in mobilizing state and local resources.

It is widely acknowledged that, despite increased Social Security benefits, the retirement income crisis affecting millions of
elderly persons remains unsolved. Year after year, public documents, reports, and studies are filled with the same finding: The
root problem affecting older Americans is inadequate income to
support their major expenditures—housing (typically accounting
for one third of their budgets), food, and medical care. Serious
gaps exist between what is funded by the Older Americans Act and
these critical needs of the aged, and this remains true even of the
most promising of the act's programs, namely, the Community
Service Employment Program. In 1975, when the Older American
Community Service Employment Act was incorporated into the
Older Americans Act as Title IX, it was operating at an annual
level of $36.4 million and 12,400 job slots. In spite of increased
funding for fiscal year 1976, little program expansion occurred
because of inflation and minimum wage increases; the number of
job slots during fiscal year 1975 was maintained at 12,400, a number that represented roughly 0.3 percent of the potentially eligible population (U.S. House, 1976, p. 412). Congress raised fund-

ing from $90.6 million in July, 1977 to $190.4 million in July, 1978, increasing the number of jobs to 47,000. President Carter's 1979 budget request of $228.45 million provided for no program expansion; rather, the fiscal year 1978 job slots at 47,000 were simply retained. Obviously this number of jobs represents only a fraction of the millions of older Americans who could and would work if provided the opportunity. At current levels less than one percent of the 5.4 million eligible older Americans are provided employment in this program (U.S. House, 1977e, p. 103; and Ossofsky in U.S. House, 1978c, p. 11).

Another argument against expansion of the Older Americans Act and other age-segregated programs is that they drain the budget away from the competing needs of the younger generation (Samuelson, 1978a, b). The youth-versus-old-age controversy surfaced in the Great Society programs. It reemerged during the Nixon administration, which employed it as a rationale for its fiscal conservatism toward categorical programs and its slashes in their funding support. The argument continues to be used with little evidence to support it.

Choices Under the Older Americans Act

The Older Americans Act has restricted the means of achieving its larger objective of independent living for the elderly to planning, coordination, and services strategies. The act has imposed limits on choice and created structural mechanisms for institutionalizing those limitations. But the implementation of programs is also constrained by the dominant ways of thinking about problem solving for specific social problems (Warren, Rose, and Bergunder, 1974). The planning and coordination strategy not only reflects the dominant view of the experts on the nature of the problems, the action required to solve the problems, the methods to be used, and who will carry out the tasks, but it legitimizes the role of expertise and the status of experts. Under such a model, failures to respond to social problems are rewarded in that they may be interpreted as demonstrating the need for more, not less, of the prescribed intervention—for example, coordination. Designated agencies, such as state units and area agencies, are able to use their definitions of appropriate intervention strategies to retain bureaucratic control.

Because organizations are jealous of the right to control their internal workings, intervention strategies based on reforming or rearranging interorganizational relations usually are resisted vigorously and often are doomed to failure. Policies in which success is based upon interorganizational relations tend to solidify existing power relationships among organizations, to legitimize the interactions based on shared understandings, and to offer little hope for promoting innovations in the development of comprehensive service systems (Warren, Rose, and Bergunder, 1974). Organizations are likely to participate only halfheartedly in cooperative exchanges and in any necessary reordering to accomplish innovative changes because they fear loss of autonomy through such activities.

Success of program implementation depends on the reasonable probability that critical actors will cooperate. The pooling and coordination strategy in the Older Americans Act creates the very difficult requirement of obtaining the voluntary cooperation of totally independent organizational units in the absence of political and economic incentives. In programs where officials have responsibility for program coordination, the mandate essentially is to clear their policies, programs, or activities with other officials who have a stake in the issue. How to do this—by coercion, bargaining, exerting power, and/or securing consent—is the question. In the words of Pressman and Wildavsky: "Telling another person to coordinate . . . does not tell him what to do. . . . Everyone wants coordination—on his own terms. Invocation of coordination does not necessarily provide either a statement of, or a solution to, the problem, but it may be a way of avoiding both when accurate prescription would be too painful. . . . Coordination means getting what you do not have. It means creating unity in a city that is not unified" (1973, p. 134).

In the multiple-dimensional strategy of the Older Americans Act, which depends on the voluntary participation of a large and complex group of organizational actors, there can be little precision in predicting the consequences of one's actions. The inability to learn from experience also results from the disparity between the design and implementation features of the Older Americans Act. After the program is designed and the funds appropriated, program implementation is left to agency administrators and program managers, with little attention from those who designed the programs or those who enacted the legislation. The result is often failure.

Implementation problems are most likely to occur in broad, multiple-aim programs that require extremely complex, highly uncertain, and often contradictory implementation processes for accomplishment. For coordination policies in particular, the requirement of joint action extends the number of relevant actors and decision points, increasing the unpredictability of action and decreasing the probability of program success. Perhaps most important, policy failures are easily attributed to implementation failures and weaknesses in the agencies and actors responsible for implementation rather than to mismatches between ends and means in the policy design. The confounding of design and implementation obscures the real reasons for policy failures, which in the case of coordination lie not in the implementation difficulties (which genuinely do exist) but in the inappropriateness of coordination to the cause of the problem—social inequality. Such difficulties existed in the Economic Opportunity and the Economic Development acts, and they are present in the Older Americans Act as well.

In the years between 1963 and 1965 the "problem" of the elderly was defined as: (1) fragmentation of federal programs for the aged, with a resulting lack of direction and coordination; (2) lack of visibility and meaningful representation of the elderly within the government; (3) the need to replace the pervasive welfare ideology with the programmatic concept of the rights of the aged; (4) the absence of trained manpower and gerontological expertise to develop services for the elderly; and (5) lack of empirical research to provide solutions in the problematic areas of health, income, and housing. The 1965 Older Americans Act offered a solution to these problems, first, by establishing an agency within the federal bureaucratic structure that would simultaneously provide access to high-level officials and give visibility to the problem;

and, second, by providing federal dollars for gerontological train-ing and for research and demonstration projects to yield empirical understanding of the problem and possible solutions.

More than a decade later, the "problem" continues to be viewed primarily as one of organization and technical manage-ment, resolvable by technocrats, planners, and administrators (U. S. House, 1977a). Organizationally, the thrust has been seeking ad-vancement of the status and authority of the Administration on Aging within the federal bureaucracy and thus helping to carry out its difficult mandate of coordinating federal programs affecting the elderly. The solution to management issues is perceived as re-quiring more experts and technology. A primary assumption is that access for the elderly to social and health benefits would be relatively nonproblematic "if only" barriers to coordination were dismantled by the application of better planning methods, com-puterized technology, or more money for research, demonstration, and coordination.

Not surprisingly, a few voices representing the elderly them-selves have repeatedly testified that their "problem" is a level of income inadequate to meet their essential needs in health, housing, and transportation. Maggie Kuhn, national convenor of the Gray Panthers, has observed that older persons have no voice in plan-ning and decision making; she emphasized the alienation experi-enced by older people in combating a system that deals with only fragmented, specialized parts of a person's life rather than the whole person. For the elderly themselves, the problem is both po-litical and economic, while for those clearly benefiting from the aging network, the problem is primarily one of management, administration, and planning, in which little (if any) consideration is given to the structural conditions that necessitate the creation of social services in the first place.

Federal and state programs cannot effectively use coordi-nation as a means of controlling costs because of the interests that benefit from a bureaucratic, uncoordinated, and fragmented ser-vice system (Friedland, Alford, and Piven, 1977). Decentralization and the resulting bureaucratic autonomy and fragmentation of political authority impede government capacity to act. Fragmentation works against large heterogeneous groups, such as the aged, that possess few resources, and it augments the influence of specialized dominant interests on government policies, "facilitating the private control of public power in a manner that has depoliticized decision making and has insulated it from partisan electoral controls" (Alford and Friedland, 1975, p. 452).

Why does the Older Americans Act follow a course similar to that already tried unsuccessfully for other social problems? In spite of its known weaknesses, why does the comprehensive planning and coordination strategy receive increasing support as a mechanism for redressing urban social problems? Warren (1973b) has observed that this strategy is functional in a number of respects: it legitimates and reinforces social agencies at a time when they are under attack for their ineffectiveness in addressing social problems; it serves the viability and expansion needs of these agencies by defining the solution to social problems in terms of a services strategy; and it provides a rationale and support for the important growth industry composed of social science and professional practitioners. Perhaps most significant, the planning and coordination strategy with its service focus permits the larger deficiencies of the social system to be ignored, thus contributing to the maintenance of existing class, status, and power distributions in the population (Estes, 1976c, p. 315). It functions, as Rose has observed, "to extend the control of institutions over the lives of their victims by legitimating the participation of these institutions in the 'solution' of problems defined to exclude the role of the economic and political structures" (1971, p. 26).

Thus, social intervention strategies that require interorganizational relations for their implementation provide a protective buffer against threatening change and act as a constraint on organizations that might otherwise initiate substantive changes. Both innovation and responsiveness are easily blunted in the interrelationships of aging network organizations, although their coordination activities legitimate their continuing effort. Warren's interorganizational studies conclude that coordination occurs through marginal changes that in no way attack the core problems of structured inequality (Warren, Rose, and Bergunder, 1974). These limitations of coordination as a policy strategy at least partially explain why one consequence of the area planning and social services strategy of the Older Americans Act appears to be a failure even in reducing the fragmentation of services.

Finally, goal displacement may have multiple consequences. In an earlier study of planning agencies for the elderly, I found that their activities often served the primary purposes of: (1) labeling the problem of the aged as a social problem of consequence in the local community; (2) advancing work in the field of aging as a legitimate profession (with or without a practicing knowledge base); (3) developing and presenting for public acceptance the planners as core experts in the field of aging; and (4) attempting to secure the recognition that would enable these professionals to influence future planning or other community activities in the field of aging (Estes, 1974b). These interests took precedence over concerns with expanding services. There is little in the creation of area agencies on aging to counteract the continuance of such goal displacement problems.

The same implementation issues continue to plague the area planning and social services strategy: centralization versus decentralization, planning versus politics, institutional change versus direct service delivery, and broad mandates and ill-defined target groups versus categorical programs with clearly specified eligibility requirements. Throughout the past two decades there have been various attempts to forge a new social policy for government intervention. The relative success or failure of the Economic Opportunity Act, revenue sharing, and the Social Security Act's new Title XX have important implications for the future. The most important point in this analysis is that reforming the area planning strategy, that is, attempting to fine tune it, will prove ineffective. Problems of implementation inhere in its design; as Benedict (1978) and others have pointed out, what is needed is a new national perspective on the alternative program designs that could be used to address the problem of inappropriate institutionalization and independent maintenance of our nation's elders.

Such a new perspective, however, faces the great obstacles that reside in the pluralistic aspects of our government, wherein interest groups joust for advantages in the aging enterprise. Often these groups make compromises by incorporating intentional ambiguities in statements of goals and strategies in order to protect their freedom to seek further advantages. An examination of pluralism, intentional ambiguity, and interest-group politics may suggest a new national perspective on age-determined interests and the appropriate program design to meet the needs of an aging population.

IV

Pluralism,
Interest-Group Politics,
and Policy Ambiguity

═══════◯▭◯═══════◯▭◯═══════

The classical theory of pluralism . . . portrays the system as a balance of power among overlapping economic, religious, ethnic, and geographical groupings. . . . As ideal, the system is celebrated because . . . [it] . . . promotes . . . a plurality of laudable private and public ends. . . . On this view, the conventional pluralist interpretation is not so much wrong as it is systematically misleading. For conventional pluralist theory focuses on the competition of elites . . . while the critics believe that a more accurate picture results when one examines the biased context . . . within which elite competition occurs [Connolly, 1969, pp. 3, 13].

Implementation issues and possible policy alternatives cannot be adequately examined without consideration of the political process that created and sustains the Older Americans Act. Direct causes for the failure of that act are the importance of the ideology of pluralism in the political process, the role and influence that pluralism provides for special interests, and the ambiguous legislative mandates that permit continued special-interest influence in all processes of implementation. Although initially enacted during an unusual period of activism in modern American political history,

61

the Older Americans Act has nonetheless been shaped by the same attitudes, values, interests, and political and economic forces that dominate many policy decisions. And just as other domestic social programs initiated in the mid 1960s have fallen victim to the power of special interests, so has the Older Americans Act. Let me try, then, to describe the political context within which the future of the aging enterprise will be shaped by answering these questions: How has the ideology of pluralism affected the Older Americans Act? What is intentional ambiguity, and how has this been used in both the legislative mandates of the act and in its implementation? What is the role of special interests, and why are they becoming the dominant force in the aging enterprise?

Pluralism

The ideology of pluralism is an important element in American politics and is inherent in the public's perception of how democracy functions. But I find three major inadequacies in this classic theory: (1) it equates organized representation and interest-group participation with democratic participation of the individual citizen, thereby nullifying the significance of individual (in preference to group) action; (2) it fosters the belief that equal access is provided all relevant parties through interest-group politics and ignores the fact that citizens with important concerns, but who are not organized, are excluded from the political process; and (3) it assumes the existence of an underlying value consensus that will make whatever results from the competitive interplay of organized interests congruent within broad areas of value agreement. This view is supported by Dahl (1956), but it sharply contrasts with the assumptions about the social construction of reality employed here.

In contrast to the tenets of pluralistic theory, one premise of this book is that the ideology inadequately explains how social policy, its content, and its consequences are developed. Policies derived from bargaining among interest groups cannot be assumed to be the product of open and fair competition, nor can it be assumed to represent the larger public good. Although policy questions may invoke the competitive interplay of different interests, policies result from structural interests and serve them. The term *structural interest* refers here to built-in social interests that "do not have to be organized in order to be served" (Alford, 1976, p. 14). Policies tend to reflect and support the dominant social and economic interests in society. Because structural interests are served by a society's major legal and social institutions, they do not have to continuously act to defend themselves. Others do that for them. Businesses, service providers, social planners, and professionals are among the structural interests that may be dominant in one or another policy. Serious competition over policies may exist among interest groups, but such conflicts are likely to be over who gets what share of a program or an appropriation. Competition of this kind in no way challenges the underlying understandings, operations, and power configurations of society. This pattern has certainly characterized the Older Americans Act since its inception. As the interest groups composed primarily of providers, professionals, and planners expanded, there was rarely a challenge to the basic assumptions of the Older Americans Act, only support for an expansion of the program, with competition primarily over who should get what amount of the dollars appropriated.

While pluralist theory is accurate in describing politics in terms of competing interests, it is misleading in that it ignores "the biased context or the 'other face of power' within which elite competition occurs" (Connolly, 1969, p. 13). As C. Wright Mills noted, "the goals for which the interests struggle are not merely given; they reflect the current state of expectation and acceptance" (1956, p. 246). These expectations are socially constructed versions of what may be appropriately treated as individual, private troubles or as public issues. The widely accepted imagery of American pluralism has provided an important rationale for the increasing involvement of private organizations in public policy determination. Some critics of pluralism argue that the primary function of the federal government has been transformed from active decision making to the more passive facilitation of conflict resolution among interest groups. Concerned by this entrenchment and by the accompanying legitimation of interest-group bargaining in public policy, Lowi argues that our society now must strive for "freedom from association" in order to prevent interest-group politics from converting "rule of law" into "policy without law." In essence, the latter is the same as "rule by delegation," in which change-oriented goals are likely to be transposed into "negotiable and administrable goals" that preserve the existing order (1971, pp. 57–60).

The democratic, consensual view of interest-group politics, which is the ideology of pluralism, provides support for a corollary theme of American politics—decentralization. Both the delegation of power to local government and the broad discretionary authority that usually accompanies it are consistent with a theory of politics that presumes a minimal need for government priorities or intervention to ensure a democratic and fair representation of the public interest in policy making. In contrast to this more sanguine view, I think that decentralization is both cause and effect of intentional ambiguity—the ramifications of which are crucial for understanding the aging enterprise.

The Older Americans Act, the Model Cities Act, the Economic Opportunity Act, the 1967 Comprehensive Health Planning and Public Health Service Amendments, and the 1972 State and Local Fiscal Assistance Act have all incorporated the principles of decentralization and discretion (autonomy) in setting and implementing program priority. They are (or were) based on ambiguous legislative mandates, including decentralization policies that granted broad governmental authority to administrators who were not directly accountable to an electorate. Because of this, they are able, in Lowi's terms, to make "policy without law." In such cases, particularly when the legislative or administrative mandate is ambiguous and highly discretionary, the tendency is for the policy to become whatever emerges from administrative perspectives and/or interorganizational, interest-group bargaining. Under these circumstances, there is no assurance that such policies will be consistent throughout states and localities or that they will be equitable and responsive to the needs of the people to be served.

What may occur instead is the objectification and institutionalization of ad hoc decisions made by administrators and other involved interests (Berger and Luckmann, 1966). Many of these policies are simply immediate responses to momentary situations for which long-range, unintended consequences are not anticipated. Staff are loath to acknowledge the casual and nonobjective bases of many of their decisions and actions, for to do so might diminish their discretionary authority. Thus, unplanned and momentary responses are likely to be institutionalized as concrete and objective formulations of the intended policies. In addition, and perhaps most importantly, such policies without law result in an abrogation of citizens' rights, because those who construct policies through these practices neither have mandates from the public nor are they accountable to it.

Decentralization, discretion, and ambiguity serve organized interests. In providing broad delegations of authority, government policies can be converted into programs and resources that serve the most powerful interest groups and those that are institutionally located close to sources of power. The bargaining among organized interests that ultimately defines and delimits issues and policies works to the advantage of highly organized, well-funded interests.

In the case of the Older Americans Act, area agencies on aging perform as the primary interest groups in negotiating the coordination and planning of services for the elderly. Current policy largely protects the implementation process from public interference because most of the action is emergent; that is, it is not specified in advance. In the area planning and social services programs, both task and goal determination are accomplished through interest-group bargaining, which politicizes program implementation and deflects energies from the delivery of services. Because of the broad and vaguely formulated delegations of agency authority, agency implementers must negotiate the content and process of actual program enactment with all participants. Thus, an implementing agency, such as an area agency, must "plug into the group process" (Lowi, 1971, p. 59) in order to carry out its assigned tasks. The potentially deleterious consequences of broad delegations of authority to interest-group government have led Lowi (1971) to propose that the Supreme Court be asked to declare them unconstitutional. Such a mandate, he argues, perhaps could be the most important revolutionary force available to the public.

Intentional Ambiguity

The general problem of intentional ambiguity, a term employed here to denote legislative and administrative mandates that are deliberately vague and nonspecific, is characteristic of the Older Americans Act, as well as of many other domestic social programs. By being general, policies may provide discretion, latitude, and permissiveness in determining program goals, clientele, emphases or strategies within programs, specific services within a general policy, and processes of implementation. Intentional ambiguity is likely to characterize legislation or program implementation when (1) there is little apparent national consensus on the nature of the problem to be addressed, the goals to be achieved, or the methods to be used in implementing policies; (2) suggested alternative policies are thought to be politically controversial, making it risky to establish an unambiguous policy choice; or (3) a measure passed by one political party is then implemented during the administration of another party with differing policies and priorities.

Intentional ambiguity obviates the necessity for making value decisions explicit, and it permits multiple interpretations of everything that it leaves ambiguous. Thus, because of the breadth and vagueness of major aspects of the Older Americans Act, as well as the contradicting theories that underlie the policy alternatives in the act, the Administration on Aging has been required to define, redefine, and clarify the meaning and intent of the many ambiguities in this enactment. As a result, the administering agencies have had to make literally hundreds of nonpublic decisions—many of which have serious consequences in terms of who gets what.

A flood of issuances from the Administration on Aging has also been necessitated by the fact that interest groups have interpreted the act at different jurisdictional levels and from different organizational perspectives. The legislative and administrative ambiguity surrounding the act encourages different groups to interpret its language in ways that are likely to further their own goals and expand their domains, thus creating both uncertainty and conflict. The ambiguity of the act has necessitated more and more bureaucratic clarification and has increasingly shifted policy making to agency staff, who are not publicly visible and thus not directly accountable to the public in their actions. Another byproduct of the act's ambiguity has been a growing preoccupation with the bureaucratic details of implementation. This may well be at the expense of activities that might more directly benefit the aged.

Those who are most powerless in the situations created by ambiguous mandates are the program clientele, who possess the least means to redress program faults because there are no clear expectations of what are to be the actual benefits and no standards against which to measure performance. For example, the ambiguity about what coordination and pooling are allows agencies variable performances, some of which may contribute little to the aged. Also, there is small opportunity for participation by consumer constituencies in the routine problem-solving activities of the agencies that actually determine program practice, policies, and priorities.

The vagueness of public understanding of what agencies should accomplish, of what program priorities are to be, and even of who their appropriate clients are prevents the formation of solid opposition to what the agencies do, no matter what they do. Under the Older Americans Act, for example, coordination and pooling form the bedrock of the social services strategy. But the wide range of choices about what these activities are, how they are to be carried out, and what is to be accomplished by them is in no way controlled by legislative specificity enabling public accountability.

The ambiguity of the Older Americans Act makes it impossible to ensure that bureaucratic action will be congruent with legislative intent, and it serves the expansionary needs of the professions and organizations that have become accomplished in teasing out the intent of its ambiguous mandates. It also provides key actors opportunities for dramatizing certain aspects of the "aging problem" in political pressure tactics to increase resources, without having to demonstrate accomplishment (for there are no clear expectations against which to measure it).

There is a tendency to "define ambiguous situations by focusing on one part of them" (Edelman, 1977, p. 16). Thus, the Older Americans Act defines the problems of aging as endemically related to fragmentation of services. By resolving the ambiguity with a diagnosed problem (fragmentation) and a prescribed solution (planning and coordination), the act reassures the public that something is being done for the aged. In similarly assuring that nothing more drastic (for example, economic redistribution) needs to be done, the ambiguous language of the act contributes to the maintenance of the existing social order.

A major old age issue characterized by statutory ambiguity is the targeting of resources to the disadvantaged elderly, including minorities and the poor. The basic unresolved question here is whether the focus of the Older Americans Act should be placed equally on all old people who need services or whether resources should be targeted to those with the greatest needs. This issue is not new. The rationale for passage of the act was that it was a program for all elderly citizens. During the period from 1964 to 1966, it was clearly stated that the intent of the act was to meet the broad and generalized needs of all the elderly. This rhetoric apparently staved off Washington critics who questioned the potential overlapping of the act with Office of Economic Opportunity (OEO) legislation. Frequently, when the Older Americans Act came under attack, testimony in its defense emphasized that the act was for all the elderly, whereas other federal programs were for specific targeted groups and often imposed financial means testing to determine eligibility. Following a similar line, the Administration on Aging sought to distinguish its programs from the War on Poverty strategy. Although it seemed reasonable to many that responsibility for the poor should reside within OEO, the 1964 Economic Opportunity Act had a broad mandate that did not single out the low-income elderly. It is true that a 1965 amendment was added that stated, somewhat ambiguously, that "it is the intention of Congress that whenever feasible the special problems of the elderly poor shall be considered" (Economic Opportunity Act, 1965). The amendment did not say, however, that this responsibility ought to reside within the newly established Administration on Aging or that the Older Americans Act itself should address the needs of the elderly poor to the extent that it would limit services to other older persons.

This issue has reemerged in several recent hearings (U.S. House, 1977d; U.S. House, 1978a; U.S. Senate, 1978a). Although there is general agreement that the Older Americans Act intends to address the special needs of low-income and minority older persons, many witnesses at congressional hearings have testified that the ambiguous and discretionary language of the act is a major obstacle to implementing this intent and that the performance of state and area agencies has been extremely variable. A report on these policy issues submitted to the Federal Council on Aging in the spring of 1978 presented a detailed analysis of the problems confronting the minority elderly and the structural constraints upon program implementation (Human Resources Corporation, 1978). Thus, while the statute seemingly requires service priority to the elderly with the greatest economic and social needs, Health, Education and Welfare (HEW) regulations also "provide that an area agency on aging can avoid meeting this service priority if it is infeasible to do so" (National Senior Citizens Law Center in U.S. Senate, 1978a, p. 9). In reauthorization hearings, a National Senior Citizens Law Center representative pinpointed the problem: "The failure within the [Older Americans] Act to consistently specify service preference for those elderly Americans in the greatest social and economic need has no doubt been, in part, the [reason why HEW has issued] regulations regarding Older American Act programming which both provide for and dilute the emphasis to be placed upon serving minority and low-income older Americans" (U.S. Senate, 1978a, p. 5).

A continuing issue—and one of the principal areas of ambiguity for the area agencies—is precisely what the so-called area plans are supposed to accomplish. What do planning, pooling, and coordination really have to do with the aged? Why are pooling and coordination defined by federal regulations as social services, when their funds usually support core agency staff who are charged with responsibilities for pooling and coordination, instead of providing direct services to the aged? How is it that area planning is so easily misunderstood, as it seems to be by many of the elderly persons whom it is intended to aid? I have heard older people ask, "If area planning is so difficult to comprehend, how can you implement it?" And, "How does it relate to me?" Translated into bureaucratic language, some of their other questions might sound like this: "Aren't critical ambiguities, contradictions, and trade-offs embodied right in the act and in the structural inadequacies of the area agencies on aging? For that matter, how can the area agencies even begin to perform all their designated responsibilities, particularly under conditions of shrinking resources for social services?"

Although the planning, pooling, and coordination approach sounds like a rational one, there is continuing confusion about what area agencies do, perhaps because the result of their efforts is likely to be intangible, nonmeasurable, and of little direct relevance to the daily lives of older Americans. A plaintive hope remains that these activities may indeed help to improve the lives of the aged; whatever planning, pooling, and coordination are, they are somehow, however vaguely and variably, beneficial. Such assumptions contribute to the systematic discounting of our own personal experiences of frustration and disappointment when we see how planning, pooling, and coordination actually fail to alleviate the grief, the deprivation, the suffering, and the loneliness of the aged.

Any legislation that may be so broadly misunderstood by so many people and that is so consistently subject to multiple interpretations provides a hiding place for multiple agency and professional agendas, many of which may be different from those of the aged themselves. What this aspect of the act does, of course, is provide for the control and domination of programs and funds for the aged by experts, that is, by those planners, coordinators, and "poolers" employed by area agencies and legitimated by the Administration on Aging. As long as policies are nonspecific and ambiguous, the American "pluralist democratic" system is permitted to operate in the interest of the strongest of those who influence legislation and program operations. To date, the primary focus has not been on the aged themselves. Outcomes are rather the net result of the negotiation among interested, vested, organized, and legitimated network participants.

My discussions with congressmen and legislative staff during the last few years have revealed their disinclination either to further specify the meaning of planning, pooling, and coordination or to consider their removal from the area planning and social services program. In spite of disillusionment and continuing concern, legislators are reluctant to push for specification. They fear the unpopularity that would result from circumscribing the interest-group politics now accommodated by the ambiguous and discretionary language of the act. To challenge the planning, pooling, and coordination paradigm would be to attack the official definition of the problem as one of fragmented services. Such a challenge would also raise the awkward question of what other government policy could be substituted at a time when there will almost certainly be no additional federal appropriations to make possible new definitions of the problem.

Binstock and Levin (1976) argue that one reason for congressional reluctance to specify "substantive issues of policy implementation" is that this nonspecification provides a circuit breaker for coping with the "overload of popular demands for adopting policies of social intervention" (p. 519). This circuit-breaker legislative pattern often results in the definition of "the substantive responsibilities of these implementing entities . . . in the most general of terms . . . and a flexible, competitive process . . . established for distributing funds to organizations that are directly engaged in operating programs" (p. 519).

The nagging doubts about the planning, pooling, coordination strategy have resulted in the development of the services strategy. First, the 1972 nutrition program was enacted as a direct service program prior to the 1973 amendments, which created area agencies on aging and the institutional change strategy. In 1975 priority service requirements were added to assure funding by area agencies of four specific social services with a minimum percentage of their allocated resources. Recent amendments to the Older Americans Act contain a provision that a fixed percent of area agency funds must be spent on either legal services, access services, or home health services.

Ultimately, of course, the question arises of where older people are left, after all the debates and struggles over programs and legislation. In particular, what will be the effect of the ambiguities in the Older Americans Act? Hudson's recent observations do not engender optimism about the probable benefits of ambiguous mandates. In his study of Title XX of the Social Security Act, he concludes that this legislation is permissive in that the choices of goals and service emphases, as well as the methods of carrying them out, occur in the implementation process rather than in the legislation. The permissiveness in the Title XX case is characterized by (1) general and abstract goal statements, (2) discretion for administrative officials, (3) variation in the particulars of implementation, and (4) open administration that encourages inputs from interested parties. The result, Hudson reported, is that there is "good reason to expect that goals and services will not accurately reflect the incidence of service needs in the states" (1977, p. 42).

In answering the question of why services are not directed to those in greatest need, Hudson notes: "For services to be allocated in proportion to need requires that the incidence of needs be known, the resources of different actors be proportional to need, and that the conditions of need be the dominant criterion which determines the way . . . actors employ their resources" (p. 42). He also noted that Title XX services are likely to be "tailored toward the existing service structure" rather than vice versa, because "professional/provider/advocate groups will . . . seek funding for the services with which they are most closely identified and which they will be able to offer with the least organizational disruption" (p. 42). He found that, with the exception of a stated requirement for Aid for Dependent Children and Special Supplementary Income recipients under Title II, there is little legal leverage within the Social Security Act to assist those with the most severe or intractable problems. The absence of incentives in the programs are such that the needs of these people are not likely to be adequately addressed.

My joint study of accountability under the Older Americans Act for the U.S. Senate Special Committee on Aging attests to the permissive nature of the Older Americans Act and the discretion that it affords administrative agencies and their interorganizational partners in the choice of goals, services, and implementation processes (Estes and Noble, 1978). This raises the question of whether the Older Americans Act is likely to be any more responsive than Title XX to the most needy.

Interest-Group Policies

Compounding the problems associated with intentional ambiguity and permissive legislative enactments are the interest-group politics fostered by the Older Americans Act and the multiple agencies it has created. Area agencies on aging are meant to act as interest-group advocates for the aged. One major consequence of the Older Americans Act has been the creation of more than 3,500 state and area agencies and service providers, which have been drawn into extensive interorganizational relations and competition with one another and with other agencies—both within and among governmental levels. It is the agencies and providers funded by the Administration on Aging that comprise what former U.S. Commissioner Arthur Flemming first labeled the aging network.

In the sense that the Older Americans Act has directly and indirectly created a network of planning and provider agencies and professional organizations, it has been possibly the single most influential catalyst to interest-group politics in the field of aging. To date, there have appeared at least three national trade associations—the National Association of State Units on Aging, the National Association of Area Agencies, and the National Association of Nutrition Directors—and a number of special centers devoted to specific minority concerns; for example, the National Center for the Black Aged, the Asociación Nacional Pro Personas Mayores, and the National Indian Council on Aging. In addition, the Administration on Aging has supported multiple university- and college-based gerontology programs that have created their own national association, the Association for Gerontology in Higher Education.

All of these newer organizations have, for one reason or another, collaborated on specific issues with one or more of the established membership organizations (for example, the American Association of Retired Persons and the National Council of Senior Citizens) and the trade associations of professionals, including such providers as the American Association of Homes for the Aging and the National Institute of Senior Centers. Between 1977 and 1978 this organizational proliferation culminated in the creation of two ad hoc national coalitions on aging—one of senior organizations and the other of leaders in the field of aging. Their efforts have been aimed primarily at increasing the Carter administration's commitments to the field. Each of these organizations claims official and expert status with regard to the problems of the aged. To the degree that these organizations and coalitions are organized and funded, they are able to act as the entrepreneurs of old age policies in the United States.

The agencies created, nurtured, and legitimated by the Older Americans Act—primarily area planning agencies, senior centers, nutrition agencies, and their national associations—have become the focus of government policy for the aged. Older Americans themselves have been relegated to the background. Predictably, these agencies have taken on a momentum of their own, demonstrating the primacy of organizational tendencies toward survival, maintenance, and enhancement (Estes, 1973; 1974b). This pattern is not limited to the field of aging but is evident throughout American government. Government sponsorship and facilitation of the efforts of organized interest groups is an important part of contemporary American politics. Contrary to the ideology of pluralism, however, it is a politics without equal access for all citizens.

The Older Americans Act is an important example of interest-group liberalism (Lowi, 1969; Binstock, 1971) wherein Older Americans Act agencies, enjoying official status, define, validate, and institutionalize the problems of the aged. In a most blatant and tragic form, the needs of the aged are replaced by the needs of the agencies formed to serve the aged, and this transposition turns the solution into the problem. This is not to deny that area agencies and other organizational units created by the Older Americans Act have made important, visible, and in many cases, direct gains for the elderly. Rather, it is to say that the interests of the aged, as perceived by the aged themselves, are not institutionalized as guiding principles of the act. As recently described by Health, Education, and Welfare Secretary Califano, interest-group politics are of growing concern to observers of the national political scene. "I think we have reached the point where the greatest builder of bureaucracy in the world today is the U.S. Congress. And Congress is doing it because it wants to help the narrow interest groups that feel they could not otherwise be protected" ("The Beneficent Monster," 1978). President Carter somewhat later reemphasized the power of the special interests and their influence in Congress (*Honolulu Advertiser,* August 25, 1978).

David Broder, one of America's most distinguished political reporters, has provided a critical analysis of interest-group government and public policy: "One theory of democracy is that from the competition of these myriad special interests will evolve, through the unseen hand of the political marketplace, a set of decisions, of priorities, that somehow add up to the national interest. Frankly,

I do not think that is likely. Everything I have seen in covering Washington over the past four administrations points to a contrary conclusion. There is no 'free market' in the political influence game. Some interests are far more powerful than others, so powerful that they can almost rig the game to assure a favorable outcome to themselves" (1972, p. 173). He goes on to say that "when the influence game is played as it is in Washington today, I am not willing to trust the future of my country to the unregulated, unmediated clash of interest groups" (p. 174). His solution is to revitalize the major political parties, to strengthen party government, and to stimulate active citizen participation in the political process at all levels of government. Because of the fundamental and systemic nature of the problems facing the United States, he believes that only through broad citizen participation, rather than interest-group politics, can the problems be dealt with. Broder sums it up this way: "If we do nothing, we guarantee our nation will be nothing. There is nothing for nothing anymore. Our choice is simple: either we become partakers in the government or we forsake the American future" (p. 265).

The dominance of interest-group bargaining in determining social policies for the United States has had profound consequences for the aged. The Older Americans Act, the Administration on Aging, and state units and area agencies on aging are but examples of this overwhelming force in American politics. Will it be possible to reverse this process? Can party government and citizen participation effectively counter the powerful interest-group forces? It is clear to me that only when the pluralistic model of private interest-group bargaining is abandoned as the major vehicle for deciding government policy for the aged will the broader public interest and the authentic interests of the aged be likely to assert significant influence on aging policies. This will require circumscribing the latitude presently provided and implementing authority by abandoning the intentional ambiguity that characterizes most social legislation for the aged.

Philip R. Lee
Carroll L. Estes

V

Eighty Federal Programs for the Elderly

When an older person has a need for a particular service, for example in-home health services, where can he turn for help? The answer, unfortunately, is "it all depends." Home health and supportive services are provided under Medicare, Medicaid, and the social services program under Title XX of the Social Security Act, home health demonstration grants under the Public Health Service Act, two different titles of the Older Americans Act, the Senior Companion and RSVP volunteer programs under ACTION, the Older Americans Community Service Employment program, Senior Opportunities and Services under the Community Services Act, and other statutes. All of this adds up to a bewildering maze of programs and regulations that is a nightmare for the elderly person trying to find his or her way through it [Pepper in U.S. House, 1977, p. 1].

For the past forty years, the United States has been moving toward a national aging policy. Although the present wide range of federal programs does not add up to a coherent national policy, progress has been made in understanding the source of the basic problems facing the elderly in this country and in seeking solutions to those problems. Many federal programs have evolved because of failures in the private sector to provide even minimal solutions—Social Security retirement income and Medicare are two examples. Some federal programs have affected virtually all of the elderly, while others have affected only a very few. Some programs have seemed effective, while others have failed to achieve even very limited objectives.

The lack of a coherent national aging policy is evident in the multiplicity of federal policies and programs affecting the aged. In an effort to examine the effect of these policies on the aged, we attempted to determine just how many programs are currently authorized and how effective they have been. In 1977, it was noted by the House Select Committee on Aging that "there are between 50 and 200 federal programs providing 'major assistance' to the elderly" (U.S. House, 1977b, p. 139). Among the many federal programs, the Select Committee identifies forty-seven major programs benefiting the elderly (U.S. House, 1977b). Recently, the number of programs was said to be 134 (Stanfield, 1978). We have identified at least eighty programs in the *1978 Catalog of Federal Domestic Assistance* that we believe benefit the aged directly or indirectly. The programs fall into the broad categories of cash assistance, in-kind transfers, and direct provision of goods and services. We did not examine tax policies, regulatory policies, or the employment policies of federal departments and agencies as they might affect the aged.

Most of the federal laws designed to benefit the aged reflect the ideology of pluralism and the strength of special interests. Medicare and Medicaid are particularly costly examples of the powerful influence of physicians and hospitals, as well as their allies in the health insurance and drug industries. Medicare, for instance, has done more to protect the interests of physicians, hospitals, and health insurance companies than it has to assure the aged access to decent medical care at a reasonable cost. The influence of special interests on policies for the aged is particularly serious because the aged are more vulnerable than any other group in society to the effects of public policies. Not only do the aged bear a disproportionate burden of chronic illness and disability, but most must live on low fixed incomes and suffer the special stigma imposed by American society on those who are no longer employed in full-time jobs.

The Older Americans Act spawned a variety of direct and indirect services to meet the needs of the aged. These are among the more than eighty different federal programs designed to assist the aged directly or indirectly. In addition to creating new service programs and providing a means for planning and coordination, the Older Americans Act defined a number of national goals for the aged, including an adequate income in retirement, the best possible physical and mental health, suitable housing, employment without age discrimination, and efficient community services. But what do the many federal programs actually contribute to the achievement of these goals? And how do current federal policies and programs measure up to the needs of the aged and the goals established by the Older Americans Act?

Federal policies and programs meant to serve the elderly directly or indirectly have been classified by the Select Committee on Aging, U.S. House of Representatives (U.S. House, 1977b) as follows:

• Income maintenance
• Employment and volunteer service
• Housing
• Health care
• Social service programs
• Transportation
• Training and research programs

(See Table 2.) The elderly may be eligible for the programs because of their age, because they are poor, or because they are designated as beneficiaries (for example, Social Security). They may also benefit if they live in an area served by a particular program or if they have a special problem, such as unemployment. A great deal has been made of the benefits to the aged of these numerous federal programs, as has been the case for such multibillion dollar programs as Social Security and Medicare that serve almost all of the aged, as well as for programs that serve only a small number of the aged directly, such as the Older Americans Act. Much stress is placed on expenditures as reflecting not only the magnitude of federal programs but their benefits for the aged. Health, Education, and Welfare Secretary Califano (1978) esti-

mated that federal programs would provide $122 billion in bene-
fits for the elderly in fiscal year 1978. We will demonstrate that
the lauded magnitude and expenditures of these U.S. social policies gave a grossly distorted picture of the actual benefits of these
programs, while hiding their inability to improve the condition of
the aged.

The Department of Health, Education, and Welfare (HEW)
has direct responsibility for major programs that provide cash
transfer or in-kind benefits, which paid out $94 billion for the aged
in fiscal year 1978. Two of these programs—Medicare and Medicaid—paid out funds to the providers of health services, while six
programs—Social Security Disability Insurance, Retirement Insurance, Special Benefits for Persons Aged Seventy-two and Over,
Old Age Survivors Insurance, Special Benefits for Disabled Coal
Miners ("black lung" benefits), and Supplementary Security Income—made their cash transfers directly to individuals. The great
bulk of these payments to the elderly were their earned Social Security retirement benefits. In addition to these programs $14 bil-
lion in earned benefits was paid the elderly under the federal civil
service and military retirement programs and the railroad retirement program. It was also estimated by Secretary Califano (1978)
that the federal government spends $4 billion annually on direct
social services (for example, through Title XX of the Social Security Act and Older Americans Act) and employment programs for
the elderly.

The departments and agencies that play a major role in programs for the aged, in addition to HEW, include Agriculture (food
stamps), Housing and Urban Development (housing for the elderly
and handicapped, housing subsidies), and the Veterans Administration (compensation and pensions, medical care). Others that
play a role in administering or monitoring some of the many federal programs of potential benefit to the aged include the Transportation, Labor, Energy, Treasury, and Commerce departments,
the Small Business Administration, the Community Services
Administration, ACTION, the Civil Rights Commission, and the
Civil Service Commission. The number of federal programs of
potential benefit to the aged and the level of federal expenditures

Table 2. Federal Programs Benefiting the Elderly, By Category and by Agency

Program	EXECUTIVE DEPARTMENTS																					INDEPENDENT AGENCIES		
	Agriculture		Health, Education, and Welfare								Housing and Urban Development					Labor	Transportation	Treasury						
	Farmers Home Administration	Food and Nutrition Service	Administration on Aging	Office of Education	Health Services Administration	Health Care Financing Administration	National Institute on Aging	National Institute of Mental Health	Public Health Service / Administration for	Social Security Administration	Office of Insured and Direct Loan Programs	Office of Assisted Housing	Community Planning and Development	Employment Standard Administration	Employment and Training Administration	Urban Mass Transportation	Office of Revenue Sharing / ACTION	Community Services Administration	Legal Services Corporation	Railroad Retirement Board	Small Business Administration	U.S. Civil Service Commission	Veterans Administration
Employment and Volunteer																							
Age discrimination in employment														•									
Community-based manpower programs													•										
Community service employment program for older Americans													•		•								
Employment programs for special groups													•										
Foster grandparent program																	•						
Retired senior volunteer program (RSVP)																	•						
Senior companion program																	•						
Service corps of retired executives (SCORE)																	•						
Volunteers in service to America (VISTA)																	•						
Health Care																							
Health resources development construction and modernization of facilities (Hill-Burton prog.)	•																						
Community mental health centers								•															
Construction on nursing homes and intermediate care facilities						•																	
Grants to states for medical assistance programs (Medicaid)		•																					
Program of health insurance for the aged and disabled (Medicare)		•																					
Veterans domiciliary care program																				•	•		
Veterans nursing home care program																							
Housing																							
Housing for the elderly (sec. 202)											•	•											
Low and moderate income housing (sec. 8)											•	•											

Mortgage insurance on rental housing for the elderly (sec. 231)

Rural rental housing loans

Community development

Low rent public housing

Income Maintenance

Civil service retirement

Food stamp program

Old-age, survivors insurance program (Social Security)

Railroad retirement program

Supplemental security income program

Veterans pension programs

Social Service Programs

Education programs for non-English speaking elderly

Legal services corporation

Model projects

Multipurpose senior centers

Nutrition program for the elderly

Older reader services

Revenue sharing

Senior opportunities and services

Social services for low-income persons and public assistance recipients (Title XX)

State and community programs (Title III)

Training and Research Programs

Multi-disciplinary centers of gerontology

Nursing home care, training, and research programs

Personnel training (Title IV-Older Americans Act)

Research and demonstration program (Title IV-Older Americans Act)

Research on aging process and health problems

Research on problems of the elderly (Higher Education Act)

Transportation

Capital assistance grants for use by public agencies

Capital assistance grants for use by private non-profit groups

Reduced fares

Capital and operating assistance grants

are impressive, but it is necessary to look beyond these gross statistics in order to determine how well the needs of older Americans are actually met by the eighty or more federal programs.

Income and Income Maintenance

Income and Financial Status. The Senate Special Committee on Aging has identified inadequate income in retirement as the number one problem affecting older Americans (U.S. Senate, 1978b). We concur. A host of poverty and income statistics testifies to this fact. Although families headed by individuals age sixty-five and over are not comparable in size to those under sixty-five, the differences in income are substantial. For example, the current median income of all families headed by a person sixty-five or over is 43.1 percent lower than the median income for all families. In 1976, half the families headed by an older person had incomes of less than $8,721, compared with $15,912 for families headed by a person under sixty-five, and the median income of older persons living alone or with nonrelatives was $3,945, compared with $7,030 for those under sixty-five living in similar circumstances (U.S. Senate, 1978b). In spite of the fact that the median income of the aged has more than doubled since 1965, in relation to the income of families whose head is under sixty-five, it is virtually where it was in 1950 (Clark, Kreps, and Spangler, 1978). In the 1960s there was a decline in the relative income of the aged to about 51 percent below the median income of all families, and if the aged's income is viewed only in the short-range perspective of the past ten years, there has been improvement over earlier periods.

Although the number of aged living in poverty (as technically defined) declined from 5.5 million in 1959 to 3.2 million in 1977, there was virtually no reduction in the number of elderly people living in poverty in the 1970s. Poverty, not just low income, is a fact of life for millions of the nation's elderly. The aged make up about 10 percent of the population, but they account for almost 30 percent of all persons in the United States with an annual income below $3,200. Among older Americans, over 14 percent live below the poverty line based on the revised Department of Agriculture's economy food plan that has been the basis for calculation of the poverty index in the past but that in fact underestimates the actual cost of an adequate diet and thus underestimates the actual cost of living. Using a revised estimate of food and other living costs that more accurately reflects current conditions, Orshansky calculated that the poverty-level income actually is "$4,772 for an elderly couple and $3,818 for a single individual rather than the $3,445 and $2,730 now used" (Orshansky in U.S. House, 1978g, p. 8). Using the revised poverty figures, Orshansky estimated that the current number of aged poor who have too little income to live by themselves, whether or not they are presently doing so, is not 3.3 million but 8.7 million. To maintain a modest, but adequate standard of living would require a good deal more than the poverty-level income proposed by Orshansky. The Bureau of Labor Statistics estimated that in 1976 this would require an annual income of $6,738 and that a slightly more adequate level could be maintained with an income of $10,048. It is clear that at least half of the aged did not achieve the $10,048 level of income in 1976.

Inflation has been a particular burden for the aged on relatively fixed incomes. The yearly inflation rate in the early 1960s was between 1 and 2 percent per year. In the past ten years consumer prices have almost doubled, making this the most intense period of inflation in the nation's history. The yearly inflation rate rose from less than 3 percent in 1965 to over 6 percent in 1969, then fell with the recession and price controls to about 3.5 percent for 1971 and 1972. In 1973, however, it shot up to over 8 percent and to over 12 percent the following year. After dropping to below 6 percent in 1976, it rose again and in some months of 1978 approached an annual rate of 10 percent.

The principal ways that the aged or any other group can be adversely affected by inflation have been listed by Schulz (1976): (1) assets that do not adjust with inflation may depreciate in value; (2) transfer payments for services may adjust to fee increases only with a lag; (3) earnings may lag behind price increases; (4) tax burdens may rise; and (5) since elderly persons sometimes allocate their budgets differently from others, CPI-adjusted benefits may not fully correct for increased prices. Not only have the aged suffered because the Consumer Price Index (CPI) does not reflect their cost-of-living increases but their Social Security increases are adjusted with a time lag. In addition, for the elderly homeowners in many areas, property taxes have increased rapidly and their fixed incomes have proved insufficient to meet these added costs. Although some economists disagree on the impact of inflation on the elderly (Clark, Kreps, and Spangler, 1978), we share Okun's (1970) view that the retired aged are the only major demographic group that can be identified as income losers.

In addition to the impact of inflation on the aged, the Senate Special Committee on Aging found that the aged did not share in the nation's recovery from the 1974–1975 recession. The Bureau of the Census confirmed the committee's findings and reported that although 900,000 persons under sixty-five years of age escaped from poverty in 1975 and 1976, virtually no change occurred for those sixty-five and older. The problem is particularly serious for the minority aged. The number of elderly blacks living in poverty increased by 10.3 percent, from 591,000 in 1974 to 652,000 in 1975. The number of aged among the Spanish-speaking population who were in poverty jumped by 17.1 percent, from 117,000 to 137,000. In the same period, poverty among the non-minority aged rose by 7 percent, from 2.46 million to 2.634 million. Over 36 percent of the aged blacks and 32.7 percent of the Spanish-speaking elderly were impoverished in 1975 (U.S. Senate, 1977). Unemployment was an important factor in the rise in poverty among the aged as a result of the 1974–1975 recession.

Social Security and Other Income Maintenance Programs. The great majority of the aged receive the bulk of their income from Social Security. Wages and salaries, which account for approximately 80 percent of the income of those under sixty-five, represent less than 25 percent of the income of the aged (Table 3). In 1978, out of 23.5 million elderly, fewer than 370,000 could depend on their earnings as their sole source of income. Even among this group, 46,000 (just over 12 percent) fall below the poverty level (U.S. House, 1978g). Over 16 million elderly, or 75 percent of all persons age sixty-five and over, receive no earnings from employment; most depend on Social Security, Supplementary Security Income, veterans' pensions, other government retirement benefits, or private pensions. For some, income from assets and investments is an important source of support (Table 3).

Table 3. Income of the Aged 1972–1973

Category	Average Annual Amount		
	Under 65	Over 65	Index: Under 65 equals 100
Money income before taxes	$12,702	$6,292	50
Wages and salaries	10,294	1,524	15
Self-employment	994	402	40
Social security and railroad retirement	201	2,085	1,040
Government retirement, veterans unemployment	253	450	178
Income from assets, investments, and so on	383	1,134	296
Other, including welfare; contributions, pensions, and so on	577	697	121
Personal taxes	1,978	528	27
Income after taxes	10,724	5,764	54
Other money receipts	227	188	82
Goods and services received	149	68	46
Mortgage principal paid	−358	−76	21
Net increase in assets	942	353	33
Market value of financial assets	5,490	13,511	246

Source: U.S. Senate, 1978b, p. xvii.

In 1964 there were 18 million beneficiaries of the Old Age and Survivors Insurance Program; in 1976 the number had risen to 28.4 million. Payments to these beneficiaries rose from $26.6 billion to $65.7 billion during that twelve-year period. In 1977 almost 21,722,000 elderly were receiving Social Security benefits. Of that number, 15,767,000 were retired workers, 5,789,000 were survivors of beneficiaries, and almost a quarter of a million received special benefits for persons seventy-two and over. Persons over sixty-five received approximately $71 billion in Social Security benefits in 1977 (U.S. Department of Health, Education, and Welfare, 1978). Social Security payments account for more than half of the income of 70 percent of individual beneficiaries and 50 percent of the income of elderly couple beneficiaries. Without Social Security, aptly described as "the economic backbone for the vast majority of older Americans," 60 percent of elderly families would have been poor in 1976 (U.S. Senate, 1978b, p. 19). Even with Social Security benefits, over 30 percent of the elderly were poor or close to being so by government standards. The number is reduced to 24.4 percent when other government programs (for example, food stamps) are added to the income of the aged. (See Table 4.)

The Social Security rolls have doubled since 1958. In 1977, 93 percent of the elderly were either drawing Social Security benefits or were certified to draw such benefits at retirement or at the retirement of a spouse; 30 to 35 percent of these people were also getting private pensions or retirement benefits as government workers. Another 3 percent not eligible for Social Security were eligible for other government retirement benefits—federal military and civil service pensions, railroad retirement pay, or state and local government pensions.

Although Social Security retirement benefits have increased substantially since 1965, many problems remain. Between 1965 and 1977, the monthly Social Security payment for a retired worker with a spouse rose from $127.55 per month to $366.05 per month. This is a 187 percent increase against a rise of 92 percent in the Consumer Price Index (Samuelson, 1978a, b). Between 1970 and 1977, Social Security beneficiaries received more than a half-dozen

Table 4. Distribution of Elderly Families Above and Below Poverty Level Before and After Social Insurance and Other Cash Transfers, Fiscal Year 1976

	Number of Families (in thousands)		
	Before Government Benefits	After Social Insurance	After Other Government Benefits
The poor	9,648	3,459	2,279
The near poor	722	1,471	1,658
All other	5,743	11,182	12,175
Total	16,112	16,112	16,112
	Percentage Distribution		
	Before Government Benefits	After Social Insurance	After Other Government Benefits
The poor	59.9	21.5	14.1
The near poor	4.5	9.1	10.3
All other	35.6	69.4	75.6

Source: Ball, 1978, p. 89.

increases in payments, obtaining almost a 100 percent increase during this period, yet the payments did not fully compensate for the impact of the recession, the increased unemployment among the aged, and the rapidly increasing costs of medical care, food, housing, and energy. According to Ball (1978), with the increases in 1977, average Social Security benefits were:

- $241 a month for a retired worker alone
- $400 a month for a worker and his wife (both receiving benefits)
- $223 a month for an aged widow
- $262 a month for a disabled worker
- $517 a month for a disabled worker, with wife and one or more children

Averages are only a rough measure of the benefits that are being paid, and they often conceal as much as they reveal. Of all the retirement beneficiaries, 25 percent were receiving less than $181.70, 50 percent less than $258, and 75 percent less than $318.10 a month (Ball, 1978). The annual Social Security payments received by more than 35 percent of the beneficiaries are below the poverty level of $2,720 per year. Thus, individuals who must rely on Social Security for total support have little assurance they will be able to remain above poverty-level subsistence after retirement unless their work career has been high paying and continuous enough to enable them to earn above-average Social Security entitlement and to supplement that with private pension benefits.

The failure of the current Consumer Price Index to reflect adequately the cost-of-living increases affecting the elderly poses special problems for these Social Security beneficiaries. The need for a separate Consumer Price Index has been suggested by Borzilleri (1978), who carried out a careful study of the current CPI and the most recent evidence on expenditures by the elderly. He found that prices rise faster for the elderly than is measured by the CPI. The result is lower Social Security benefits than are actually required. He found an "aggregate underadjustment of Social Security benefits in the neighborhood of $500 million over the first two-and-one-half years of operation of automatic adjustment provisions" (Borzilleri, 1978, p. 230). We fully share

Borzilleri's conclusions that the Bureau of Labor Statistics should undertake a study to determine whether or not a separate CPI for older persons should be developed and maintained.

Because of problems facing the Social Security System, including its financing and benefits, Congress enacted a major revision of the program in December 1977. Major increases in Social Security taxes will follow these revisions. President Carter's proposal to use general revenues to supplement these taxes was not accepted. We believe that Congress should reconsider the use of general revenue funds to reduce the regressive tax burden on the middle-income wage earners from their current and future Social Security taxes. This new system, which went into effect January 1, 1979, provides benefits on the basis of average indexed monthly earnings. Dollar amounts will increase in the future and benefits will be protected, at least in part, against inflation, as has been true since 1972. The Social Security cost-of-living increases may raise an elderly poor person above the level of Medicaid eligibility, thus requiring the individual to "spend down" the increases by paying more out of pocket for needed medical care. There are many individuals receiving Supplementary Security Income (SSI) benefits who, because of increased medical expenses, energy costs, and rent, actually have less disposable income than they did five years ago under Social Security and Old Age Assistance. The primary result of the 1978 Social Security amendments has been to stabilize the Social Security financing mechanisms and to assure future (not current) beneficiaries certain increments—all financed disproportionately by the middle-class wage earner. The thirty-three million people, including the twenty-two million elderly, now receiving Social Security benefits will continue to have their benefits based on actual rather than indexed earnings and there will be a five-year transitional period that will guarantee retirement benefits at least as high as the benefits of December 1978 under the old law (Ball, 1978).

The SSI program was initiated in 1974 to replace the federal-state programs of Old Age Assistance, Aid to the Blind, and Aid to the Permanently and Totally Disabled. Effective July 1977, an individual was guaranteed an income of $177.80 a month, and couples were guaranteed $266.70 a month, provided they met the income and resource tests and the other requirements of the SSI program. These income guarantees are well below the poverty level established by the federal government, which was $239 a month for an individual and $302 for a couple in 1977. The aged and disabled make up more than 95 percent of the SSI beneficiaries. In fiscal year 1978, 1.7 million aged received payments totaling $1.74 billion (Livers, 1978), the average annual expenditure per recipient thus being only about $1,000, well below subsistence levels. In New York State the average monthly benefit for the aged recipient is below the level of the previous Old Age Assistance Program. Indeed, as Zander (1978) observed, the level of relative deprivation is increasing.

Government pensions are an important source of income for the aged. Moon (1977) found that these pensions provided benefits for over 10 percent of elderly families. While the proportion of beneficiaries at the time of her analysis was about the same as it was for public assistance, the pensions provided substantially higher payments. Veterans' benefits are another source of direct financial assistance to the low-income elderly. Veterans receive compensation for service-connected disabilities without a means test, and there is an additional means-tested pension payable to the disabled, the aged, and the families of deceased veterans. The income-tested pension is only $185 a month for those with annual incomes of $300 or less and no dependents. It is only $199 a month for an aged or disabled (nonservice-connected) veteran with one dependent. In 1978, the Senate enacted amendments that would raise these pension payments above the Department of Labor's poverty index. Prior to these amendments, if a veteran had an income above $3,540 annually, he was not eligible for the pension. In 1977, 2.7 million veterans and their survivors were receiving income-tested pensions, including 538,000 veterans aged sixty-five and over. The number of elderly veterans eligible for these pensions has decreased as Social Security payments have increased, and less than 3 percent of the aged currently receive veterans' pensions. In Moon's analysis (1977) veterans' pensions and compensation (military retirement pay) per family were slightly greater than public assistance payments. Recipient families (including both pensions and compensation) comprised 9.4 percent of the total elderly population. Veterans' compensations are distributed across all income classes, while the pensions are targeted to the poor. In addition, Moon (1977) found that less than 3 percent of the aged benefited from unemployment insurance and workman's compensation and that the mean transfer payment was small. No families below the $2,000-level of income benefited from these programs. Although government pensions and, to a lesser extent, workman's compensation and unemployment insurance provide substantial benefits to some aged families, they play only a very limited role in ameliorating the economic problems of a small number of the aged.

The federal government, through SSI, now has the mechanism to abolish poverty for the elderly, blind, and disabled. The total cost of guaranteeing the poverty level of income for all three groups would be about $8 or $10 billion a year. While the eligibility requirements of the SSI program help to target the program to the poor, they also limit the program's ability to lift people from poverty status. Although the figures on the cash transfers to the elderly are impressive, it is important to recognize that almost 25 percent of elderly men and women live below or near the federal government's poverty level. It is difficult for many of the aged to survive on their Social Security or Supplementary Security incomes. The problem is compounded by the fact that federal policies penalize the thrifty and the aged person who maintains close family ties. For the SSI beneficiary, Gore has observed: "Currently whenever an individual is successful in saving expenses in one area, such savings are treated as 'income' and reduce SSI benefits. It is impossible under this system for an elderly person to ever escape from poverty" (Gore in U.S. House, 1978e, p. 4).

A case report from the National Senior Citizens Law Center dramatically illustrates the problem:

> A seventy-two-year-old woman in Iowa lost her SSI benefits entirely because the rent she doesn't pay is more than the rent she does pay. This woman rents a trailer from her son for $60.00 a month and pays $25.00 a month for the space rental. In addition, her normal expenses include $25.00 for utilities and $24.00 for $56.00 worth of food stamps. The secretary of HEW determined that her son

could rent the trailer to someone else for $150.00 a month.
The woman was assessed $90.00 in "income" for rent she
did not pay even though she was paying $85.00 a month
in rent, almost 50 percent of her total cash income. Since
her so-called "income," plus her Social Security benefits,
put her over the income limit for SSI she has had to live
on her $120.00 a month Social Security check [U.S. House,
1978e, p. 27].

The effect of present SSI policies on the institutionalized
elderly is even more restrictive. The benefit for the institutionalized elderly was frozen at twenty-five dollars per month when the
SSI program was enacted in 1974. Inflation has drastically reduced
these already meager benefits.

Although Social Security and Supplementary Security Income payments provide the bulk of the income for the aged, private pensions are of growing importance. The proportion of elderly couples with private pension income rose from 16 percent
in 1962 to 28 percent in 1976; for the single elderly retired person
the increase was from 5 to 14 percent (Samuelson, 1978b). In 1975,
private pensions paid $15 billion to 7.4 million recipients, for an
average of about $2,000 annually per recipient. Although some
major companies have adequate retirement pensions for their
hourly workers as well as their executives, Samuelson has observed
that "the private pension system suffers from three potential defects: huge variations in benefit levels, spotty coverage, and an
enormous vulnerability to inflation" (1978b, p. 1715).

Food Stamps. Food stamps have grown over the past ten years
to become one of the federal government's largest in-kind transfer
programs. In 1976 over $5.5 billion was spent on 18 million recip-
ients: the working poor, low-income Social Security beneficiaries,
and poor single adults. The elderly, however, have had a low participation rate in the food stamp program, with about only one
sixth or less of the elderly poor seeking this entitlement. Obstacles
for the aged documented by the Senate Special Committee on Aging are: (1) unawareness of the program; (2) inability or unwill-
ingness to comprehend the administrative red tape and application
procedure; (3) inability to pay the purchase price for the stamps;
and (4) the "welfare stigma" attached to the program (U.S. Senate,

1978b, p. 207). In the past, it has been difficult to determine the number of aged who have participated in the food stamp program, and it has been virtually impossible to determine the income transfer involved. In 1977, the U.S. Department of Agriculture and the Bureau of the Census analyzed data collected in a 1975 survey and determined that 1 million (6 percent) of the 17 million food stamp participants are persons sixty years of age or older, that approximately 17.9 percent of the 3.3 million elderly whose incomes are below the poverty level participate in the program, and that most households with elderly participants have zero assets. The food stamp program was not meeting the needs of the elderly poor primarily because many of them did not have thirty-five or forty dollars cash at one time to buy their way into the program. This requirement, however, was eliminated in the final version of the Food and Agriculture Act of 1977 (Public Law 95–113). Although the Carter administration proposed "cashing out" the food stamp program and providing cash instead of food stamps to needy recipients, Congress voted to continue the program.

Employment and Volunteer Service

Employment among the elderly has declined steadily for the past thirty years. In 1948, nearly half of all men sixty-five and older remained in the work force. Today only one man in five (1.8 million) and one woman in twelve (1.1 million) continue to work after age sixty-five, with employment concentrated in jobs with relatively low pay (Brotman, 1978). This significant decline in employment has been largely influenced by mandatory retirement policies, age discrimination, the availability of Social Security retirement benefits, and an economy that has rapidly applied new technologies and modes of production that afford less opportunity for older workers. Many older workers have simply been replaced by advancing technology; they have had few opportunities for training to enable them to work in this new environment. Early retirement is also a factor in the declining employment of the aged. In 1976, 75 percent of workers who applied for Social Security benefits sought the reduced benefits available to those who retire at age sixty-two to sixty-four. In 1961, only 53.6 percent of the initial applicants for retirement were under age sixty-five (Singer, 1978). After carefully examining factors that influence the labor supply of the elderly, Clark, Kreps, and Spangler noted that "there are an increasing number of studies finding that together pension systems—benefits and labor force restrictions—and health status are the most significant factors that influence the labor supply decisions of older workers" (1978, p. 931).

The Age Discrimination in Employment Act, enacted in 1967, underwent a landmark revision in 1978. Initially protecting those aged forty through sixty-four from age discrimination by most employers of twenty or more persons, and employment agencies and labor organizations with twenty-five or more members, the law was extended to include individuals aged sixty-five to seventy. The revision is applicable to workers in private employment as well as those employed by state and local governments; additional provisions (U.S. Senate, 1977) include:

- College and university faculty members with unlimited tenure can be mandatorily retired at age sixty-five until July 1, 1982, when the mandatory retirement age increases to age seventy.
- Highly paid employees with retirement benefits of $27,000 per year or more (exclusive of Social Security) can be mandatorily retired at age sixty-five.
- Mandatory retirement for most federal employees will be abolished.

Despite the potential of the new law, its short-range impact is not likely to be great. Although the Department of Labor estimated that only about 200,000 workers would continue working past age sixty-five as a result of the law, a consultant to the Senate Special Committee on Aging has estimated that the number will be 200,000 annually in the next few years (Singer, 1978).

Perhaps the most important effect of the 1978 amendments to the Age Discrimination in Employment Act will be the pressure they will exert for a national manpower policy for older workers. Such a policy should provide greater opportunity for older workers and should make it easier for them to continue in paid employment. Companies may begin to experiment with gradual retirement programs, part-time work, shared jobs, and flexible work schedules (Singer, 1978). The federal government should certainly lead the way.

Federal manpower programs, past and present, are inadequate to meet the basic needs of millions of older Americans who do not have sufficient retirement income or of those fifty-five and older who face age discrimination in the labor market. It is clear, in fact, that the United States has failed to develop a comprehensive policy to provide adequate job opportunities for middle-aged and older workers (U.S. Senate, 1977). Repeated congressional reports and hearings have documented the Department of Labor's notorious disregard of older persons and the special problems they face in the job market. For example, "In fiscal 1976, persons forty-five or older represented only 7.2 percent of all enrollees in Department of Labor manpower programs. Yet, they accounted for 19 percent of the total unemployment in October 1976. Individuals fifty-five or older represented only 2.9 percent of all enrollees in work and training programs but accounted for 8 percent of unemployment in October 1976" (U.S. Senate, 1977, p. 88). More specifically, the youth-oriented Comprehensive Employment and Training Act (CETA) has done little to meet the needs of older workers. The number of participants fifty-five and older in CETA programs under Titles I, II, and VI has hovered at a mere 5 percent and below for 1975 and 1976. In view of the less than impressive program performance of CETA, many congressmen and national organizations have fought to retain and expand the one categorical manpower program, the Community Service Employment, under the Older Americans Act. Although this program is considered to have made dramatic gains in funding, it employs less than 1 percent of the more than 5.4 million eligible older Americans (see Chapter Three and U.S. House, 1978c).

Volunteer services have long been included in federal programs for the elderly. Many of these programs, such as the Foster Grandparent Program, were initially authorized under the Older Americans Act but since 1973 have been authorized by the Domestic Volunteer Services Act and administered by ACTION and the Small Business Administration. The Foster Grandparent, Retired Senior Volunteer, and Senior Companion Programs all au-

thorize grants to public and nonprofit agencies to establish or expand volunteer service opportunities, particularly for low-income
persons who wish to give supportive services to children or adults.
These programs, as well as the Volunteers in Service to America
(VISTA), are administered by ACTION, while the Senior Corps
of Retired Executives is administered by the Small Business
Administration. Although there are now over twenty-three million
elderly Americans and millions among this group who are involved
in one or another church, community, or other volunteer service,
there are relatively few who participate in or are served by the
programs administered by ACTION.

Housing

In *Why Survive?* Butler (1975) has described accurately and
poignantly the importance of housing for the elderly:

> In human terms the issue of housing for older peo-
> ple is far more than simply providing a roof over their
> heads. When we talk about housing we are really address-
> ing the concept of 'home' and what it means to the elderly.
> The place where one lives is often profoundly connected
> with who one is and how one expresses this sense of self.
> Home is where all individuals feel most comfortable to be
> themselves, to drop social facades. Many older people also
> associate home with autonomy and control; for them it is
> sometimes the only place where they can feel certain of
> their surroundings, free from the control and restraint of
> others. Home is an expression of one's personality through
> furnishings, decorations, memorabilia, ambience, plants,
> pets. It is a familiar place in what may be a changing and
> unsteady world outside [1975, p. 101].

Information on housing for the elderly is out of date, limited in scope, and insufficient to determine the effectiveness of
various programs designed to meet the needs of the elderly. Based
on data from the 1960 census, it is likely that seven million (30 percent) of the aged live in housing that is substandard, deteriorating,
or dilapidated and scarcely inhabitable. Such housing may have no
inside toilet, no hot water for a bath or shower, and inadequate

heat in the winter (Butler, 1975). Not only are physical conditions often deplorable, but costs are often prohibitive for the elderly on fixed incomes. Housing currently represents the single most significant expenditure for the elderly, accounting for almost 29 percent of their total budget (Brotman, 1978). Rent poses special problems. Among renters seventy-five and older, rent assumes almost 50 percent of expenditures. Families with income below $5 thousand annually pay 35 percent of their income for rent, while those with an income of $15 thousand or more pay only 12 percent of their income for rent.

Elderly homeowners also have special problems: high maintenance and repair costs, rapidly rising property taxes, and skyrocketing fuel and electrical costs. For example, in Hamilton County, Ohio, the seventy-five thousand families headed by an aged individual include twenty-one thousand elderly who have difficulty meeting housing costs and upkeep payments and forty-five thousand elderly who live in homes that need repairs, as well as a significant number who live in homes that they consider dangerous (Johnson, 1978). The problem facing these people was described by Marc Johnson, manager of program development, in the Cincinnati Community Development Agency: "Many of today's elderly became homeowners during their working lives. And if the elderly citizens were black or Appalachian poor, they frequently lived in the inner cities and in the distant rural areas. Most of the elderly poor in the Cincinnati area live in the blighted inner-city areas. Displacement of the poor from the inner cities uproots the elderly and often forces them to have nowhere to go where there will be adequate quarters at the price that they are able to pay, or [where they will] be able to identify with old friends. This condition often results in the elderly moving into shameful and inadequate quarters and confining themselves to a life of endless loneliness" (Johnson, 1978, p. 2.).

If the housing problem was serious prior to the inflation, the recession, and the energy crisis of the early 1970s, problems since then have steadily increased. A few figures illustrate the rise in energy costs alone: the price of home heating oil increased 94 percent and the price of electricity increased 41.5 percent from March 1973 to March 1976; the consumer price index rose by 24 percent during approximately that same period (U.S. Senate, 1978b). The costs of maintenance, repair, and insulation have also risen rapidly in the past decade. To assist the elderly who have been hard hit by the rapid increase in energy costs, the Community Services Administration was provided $200 million for aid in the crisis that resulted from the severe winter of 1976–1977. Available for direct payment of utilities of up to $250 on behalf of individuals whose income did not exceed 125 percent of the poverty level, the funds were allocated to states under a formula based on the severity of winter, the relative costs of fuel, and the number of low-income households headed by the elderly. Program activities included weatherization, cash assistance to prevent utility cutoff, transportation, education, legal assistance, and alternate energy sources. Although the program was severely criticized as being too little, too late, short lived, and poorly managed, $200 million was again appropriated in 1977–1978. The budget request for fiscal year 1979, however, was only $10 million, a sum that unmistakably reflected the short-range nature of the government's response (Executive Office of the President, 1978).

A limited program to aid families in insulating and weatherizing their homes was initiated by the Carter administration in 1977. Authorized under the Energy Conservation and Production Act, this program provides for the purchase of materials to weatherize the homes of low-income persons, particularly the elderly and handicapped. The initial appropriation of only $27 million was allocated to forty-nine states, the District of Columbia, and Indian tribal organizations; it was anticipated that 114,000 homes could be weatherized with these funds. In 1978, $64 million was requested, an amount that would permit weatherization of approximately 220,000 additional homes. But a program of this limited scope is obviously nothing more than a symbolic gesture, not a meaningful response to a problem that affected millions of people in almost every area of the country except the Far West and the Southwest.

During the past forty years there have been six major housing programs designed to benefit the elderly: (1) Low Rent Public Housing (Housing Act of 1937, as amended); (2) Low and Moderate Income Housing (Housing Act of 1937, as amended, Section 8); (3) Rural Rental Housing Loans (Housing Act of 1949, as amended, Sections 521 and 525); (4) Housing for the Elderly (Housing Act of 1959, as amended, Section 202); (5) Mortgage Insurance on Rental Housing for the Elderly (Housing Act of 1959, as amended, Section 231); (6) Community Development Block Grant Program (Housing and Community Development Act of 1974, Title I, as amended) (U.S. House, 1977a). The Housing Act of 1937 established the first national program of low-rent public housing, and this program remains one of the major federal housing efforts to aid the poor. In fiscal year 1978 an estimated $1.8 billion was obligated for this program, making it one of the largest administered by the Department of Housing and Urban Development. But an analysis by Moon (1977) found that only 1.28 percent of all aged families benefit from the public housing program. The Housing Act of 1949 was considered a milestone because it established as a national goal a "decent home and a suitable living environment for every American family" (in Butler, 1975, p. 126). It also initiated the ill-fated urban renewal program that was to destroy many of America's central cities to provide housing for the middle and upper classes at the expense of the poor and the aged (Butler, 1975). The act also authorized a program of direct federal loans and guaranteed insurance loans for the construction or repair of rental or cooperative housing in rural areas for low-income persons, including the elderly.

The National Housing Act of 1959 authorized, under Section 202, a program of direct loans to nonprofit sponsors to develop housing for the aged and the handicapped. This program proved popular, and although only 45,000 units were built during the first decade of Section 202, it appeared to be an economical way to provide decent housing for those with special needs. In 1969 and through the early 1970s, however, the Nixon administration refused to make funds available for Section 202 programs. Instead, it substituted a loan guarantee program that increased the cost of each project substantially and benefited primarily the mortgage bankers. After a long struggle the Section 202 program was amended in 1974, and funds began to flow again in 1976. In 1977, $630 million was awarded to sponsors for the construction or rehabilitation of about 24,000 housing units. In 1978, $629.7 million was reserved for this program, $562.3 million specifically for the aged. The number of units funded for the aged was 16,900—far below the 1971 goal of 120,000 (U.S. Department of Housing and Urban Development, 1978). Even that goal is far below the need. In Los Angeles alone there are 99,000 elderly in need of housing, and there are five applicants for every available unit.

The same problem of the limited nature of these programs appears again and again. The Housing Act of 1961, the Housing and Urban Development Act of 1964, and the Demonstration Cities and Metropolitan Development Act of 1966 (Model Cities) added new authorities and programs to those already in force. The Housing and Urban Development Act of 1968 established new national housing goals, and it expanded the urban renewal, public housing, rent supplement, and Model Cities programs. The Housing and Community Development Act of 1974 attempted to apply revenue sharing and new federalism concepts to housing with little or no benefit to the elderly. But in all of these instances, the funds appropriated were far below the level needed to achieve the goals set by Congress. In 1974, the Ford administration also initiated a new program to provide rent supplements for low-income families. This program was designed to ensure that the poor would not be required to pay more than one quarter of their gross income for shelter. The initial goal of this program was to aid 400,000 families annually. But by November 1976, only 76,896 households were placed in existing units, 4,097 in new units, and 595 in rehabilitated units. Although the elderly fared reasonably well in this program, constituting approximately 44 percent of the participants, the small size of the program once again limited its effectiveness. If, then, the broadened federal housing efforts of the past few years represent an improvement on earlier efforts, they have not really reversed the damage done to the elderly by a series of forces ranging from urban renewal and highway construction to rapid rises in energy costs. For a problem of massive proportions, Congress has so far mandated only lightweight solutions.

Health, Illness, and Health Care

The aged, in the main, are in good health, although many have one or more chronic diseases. The 1975 Health Interview Survey (of the noninstitutionalized civilian population), conducted by the National Center for Health Statistics, revealed that over two thirds of the aged reported their health as good or excellent when compared with others their own age. While 22 percent reported their health as fair, only 9 percent reported their health as poor, although the proportion assessing their health as poor was twice as high among minorities (16 percent) as among whites (8 percent). (Self-assessment has been found to be an accurate reflection of health status for the aged. People who rate their health as poorer than others their age are more likely to suffer from activity-limiting chronic conditions and to use health services more often than those who report their health as good or excellent. See U.S. Department of Health, Education, and Welfare, 1977.)

Over 80 percent of the noninstitutionalized aged population reported some chronic condition in 1975, while over 50 percent of the aged poor and 40.7 percent of the nonpoor aged reported activity limitation due to chronic illness. Of those with activity limitation, 17 percent were unable to carry on their major activity. Almost 7 percent needed help in getting around, 5 percent were confined to their homes, but only 1 percent were bedridden (U.S. Department of Health, Education, and Welfare, 1977). Restricted activity days per person were twice as high for the elderly as for those under sixty-five for both the poor and the nonpoor. The poor, aged sixty-five and over, had 46.6 days of limited activity per year compared to 23.2 days for the poor under sixty-five; for the nonpoor the days of restricted activity were 31.2 and 13.7 days, respectively, for those sixty-five and over and those under sixty-five (Butler, Newacheck, and Piontkowski, 1978). Two chronic conditions caused almost half of the activity limitation among the elderly: 24 percent were restricted by heart disease and 23 percent by arthritis or rheumatism. Other conditions causing activity limitation were orthopedic impairments (11 percent), visual impairments (10 percent), hypertension (9 percent) and emphysema (8 percent of men and 2 percent of women). Old people saw physicians 50 percent more often than did those under sixty-five; they also had almost twice as many hospital stays and remained in the hospital almost twice as long as younger persons. Still, over 80 percent reported no hospitalization during the year and over 13 percent did not consult a physician. Wide variation existed in the utilization of medical care by the aged. For example, only 43 percent of the elderly reported to have arthritis had seen a physician during the year. In contrast, 80 percent of the aged with diabetes, a heart condition, or hypertension had seen a physician for their conditions within a year (U.S. Department of Health, Education, and Welfare, 1977).

The impact of this illness burden on the quality of life of the aged is enormous. Over 1 million are in nursing homes, over 3.8 million are unable to carry on their normal activities, and at least 11 million are limited in their activities. The problems increase with advancing age. Illness and disability are cited as the major reason that those sixty-five and over are unable to work. Not only does illness and disability restrict the earning capacity of the aged, but the costs of medical care drive many to a state of impoverishment. Poor health is a significant factor in accentuating and deepening the poverty of the aged; in turn, their poverty contributes to their poor health and disability. High medical care costs for the aged reflect their growing numbers, their disproportionate burden of illness, the increasing percentage who are seventy-five years old and older, and the devastating effect of price inflation during the past fifteen years. The total health bill in the United States more than tripled between 1965 and 1976, rising from $38.9 billion to $139.3 billion. Personal health care expenditures in 1976 were $120.4 billion (U.S. Senate, 1978b). The Social Security Administration estimated that 54.6 percent of the increases in personal health care expenditures between 1950 and 1976 were accounted for by price increases, 10.5 percent by population changes, and 34.9 percent by changes in the patterns and utilization of care. It has been estimated that in the past few years more than 75 percent of the increase in cost has been caused by price increases (U.S. Senate, 1978b).

The inflationary cost of health care has had its greatest impact on the elderly. Their per capita health care expenditures rose 34 percent from 1974 to 1976. In 1977, their expenses rose 14 percent ($224) to $1,745. In 1977, expenditures for those between nineteen and sixty-four were $661, and $253 for those under nineteen (Iglehart, 1978). Health care expenditures for the aged break down roughly as follows: 45 percent for hospital care, 23 percent for nursing home care, 17 percent for physician services, 8 percent for drugs, 2 percent for dental services, and 5 percent for all other items (U.S. Senate, 1978b). After the enactment of Medicare and Medicaid in 1965, public funds became an important source of funds to pay for the care of the elderly. This is particularly true for hospital care, nursing home care, and physician services. In spite of the fact that public funds pay for more than two thirds of the medical care costs of the elderly, major problems remain, particularly because of the gaps in Medicare coverage and the rapid increase in medical care costs in the past decade (Table 5).

The impact of rising costs of medical care on the elderly is strikingly evident in several statistics:

- In 1976 the aged paid $404 per capita in direct out-of-pocket medical care expenses, an amount almost equal to the total cost of their care in 1966.
- In 1976 the $404 direct per capita out-of-pocket expense was more than double the per capita out-of-pocket expense of those under sixty-five and almost equals the total cost of care of those under sixty-five ($438).
- More than 50 percent of Medicare beneficiaries spend more than $0.5 billion dollars on private health insurance premiums to fill Medicare gaps.
- Medicare beneficiaries pay $1.6 billion for the optional Part B Medicare premium.
- The aged pay out of pocket 25 percent of the nation's $10 billion drugs and drug sundries bill, although they represent only 10 percent of the population.

Medicare is the largest and most important program designed to provide the aged with access to needed medical care and protect them against the high cost of care. In 1976, 5.1 million aged had much of their inpatient hospital care covered by Medicare, and 12.7 million elderly had a portion of their physician and related services covered by Part B of Medicare. Total Medicare costs in 1976 were $17.73 billion. Although utilization is not increasing, medical care costs—and thus Medicare expenditures— are rising rapidly. Medicare expenditures rose to $20.8 billion in

Table 5. Medical Care Expenditures, 1966–1976

| | | Directly Out of Pocket | Third-Party Payments | | | |
	Total		Total	Govern-ment	Private Health Insurance	Philan-thropy and Industry
Amount:						
Under 65:						
1966	$154	$79	$75	$30	$42	$3
1976	438	153	285	127	151	7
Over 65:						
1966	446	237	209	133	71	5
1976	1,521	404	1,117	1,030	81	6
Distribution (Percent):						
Under 65:						
1966	100.0	51.1	48.9	19.4	27.3	2.2
1976	100.0	34.9	65.1	29.0	34.5	1.7
Over 65:						
1966	100.0	53.2	46.8	29.8	15.9	1.1
1976	100.0	26.5	73.5	67.7	5.4	.4

Source: U.S. Senate, 1978b, p. xix.

fiscal 1977 and were estimated to rise to $28.9 billion in fiscal 1979. Medicaid, the federally assisted and state-administered program that pays for basic medical care for the poor who are aged, blind, disabled, or members of families with dependent children, has been important for the aged. Medicaid currently provides some assistance in paying medical care bills for 21 million people. Only 18 percent (3.9 million) of these are over sixty-five, but payments to providers for their care account for 38 percent of Medicaid expenditures—a disproportion resulting from the burden of chronic illness and disability borne by the elderly and the cost of their hospital and nursing home care.

The implementation of Medicare and Medicaid in 1966 was followed by a dramatic increase in the use of hospital services but little or no increase in the use of physician services outside the hospital by the aged. Indeed, the average number of physician contacts by persons aged sixty-five and over, excluding contacts while a patient is in a hospital, nursing home, or other institution, has remained at approximately 6.6 visits per year from 1965 through 1975. (The increase in the use of physician services by the elderly poor was offset by the decrease among the nonpoor aged.) Hospital utilization, by contrast, increased sharply during the first fiscal year (1966–1967) that Medicare was implemented. The hospital discharge rate increased by 4.6 to 7.4 percent, average length of stay by 4.1 to 7.8 percent, and days of care per 1,000 elderly by 8.9 to 16.0 percent. Since then, the increase in the number of patients discharged and the decrease in the average length of stay have tended to cancel out each other so that the number of days of hospital care per 1,000 elderly people has not increased substantially (U.S. Department of Health, Education, and Welfare, 1977). Surgical rates have increased dramatically since the advent of Medicare. In 1965 there were 6,554 operations for every 100,000 people sixty-five and over; in 1975 there were 15,482 operations. Cataract surgery more than doubled, from 525 to 1,115 operations per 100,000 elderly, and arthroplasty increased from 49 to 145 operations per 100,000 elderly people. Use of prescription drugs has increased even more rapidly during this period.

Although, as noted, use of physician services outside the hospital has not increased, costs have escalated. Medicare will pay physicians a fee based on the physician's customary charges, but because of the rapid increase in physicians' fees, Medicare has raised its payments at a slower rate. And increasingly doctors have refused to accept the Medicare payment, called an *assignment*. With the growing disparity between Medicare payments and doctors' fees, more of the cost is borne directly by the elderly.

Additional problems have arisen for the elderly poor who have had to depend on state Medicaid programs as well as on Medicare. In many states the Medicaid programs have been cut back in both scope of benefits and number of individuals eligible. The federal budget for fiscal year 1979 estimated that the number of elderly receiving Medicaid benefits would decline by 97,000 (2.5 percent) for the year. This represents a decrease of 197,000 since 1977, when the elderly represented 18 percent of Medicaid recipients. This drop is due to state-initiated Medicaid cutbacks generated by state-level fiscal crises, as well as to the fact that Supplementary Security Income payments have raised some elderly poor above the financial eligibility level for Medicaid. This has created a group of elderly people highly vulnerable to the impact of medical costs because as one loses Medicaid eligibility, one loses coverage for out-of-hospital drugs and most long-term care.

The staff of the U.S. House Select Committee on Aging has analyzed the Medicaid program and has pointed out many of its serious weaknesses. Because many Medicaid benefits and policies are state determined, except in the case of federal matching funds and the establishment of minimum guidelines on the scope of services, the federal government can exert little influence. Individual states have virtual control over the scope of services offered in the Medicaid program and, to a large extent, over determining eligibility requirements as well. This problem has been summarized by the Select Committee staff: "The resultant lack of uniformity among Medicaid programs effectively varies benefit levels to the point where an impoverished elderly person in one state received as little as one third of the national average payment level" (U.S. House, 1978e, p. 52). The variations in eligibility, scope of coverage, and levels of payment for services among states results in Connecticut's Medicaid program paying providers an average of $2,709 in 1974 per aged recipient, while Alabama paid $305 and Missouri $303. Many states do not provide even the bare minimum of coverage to meet the medical care needs of the aged or other program beneficiaries.

In spite of its severe limitations, however, Medicaid plays a major role in financing long-term care, that is, medical care, home health care, social services, and nursing home and other nonhospital institutional care provided to the chronically disabled, especially the aged. Medicaid stresses nursing home care rather than the full range of services needed by the elderly. On any given day there are about 1.3 million nursing home residents in 18,300 nursing homes. Of this group, 70 percent are seventy-five years of age or older, and only 15 percent are under sixty-five. In 1975 federal, state, and local governments spent $5.7 to $5.8 billion on long-term care. Medicaid was the source of $4.3 billion (75 percent) of the total. Private expenditures totaled between $5.9 and $7.7 billion in 1975. The Congressional Budget Office has estimated that long-term care expenditures will increase from about $12 billion in

1975 to somewhere between $25.8 and $31 billion in 1980 (U.S. Congress, 1977).

The future need for long-term care relates primarily to the level of functional disability in the population, particularly the elderly. At one extreme are the severely disabled elderly who require nursing home care. These represent about 5 percent of the aged population or about 1 million people. There are millions more (probably 5 to 10 million) who could benefit from long-term care services if they were provided on a noninstitutionalized, community basis. As the population increases, the number needing long-term care services will increase to somewhere between 6 and 11 million in 1980 and between 7.4 and 12.5 million in 1985 (U.S. Congress, 1977). Among the 5 to 10 million people currently needing long-term care, an average of only about 1 to 2.7 million receive such services under government programs. In addition to Medicaid, services are provided or paid for by the Veterans Administration, Supplementary Security Income, and Title XX (social services) of the Social Security Act.

Many nursing home patients must exhaust their limited incomes and savings on nonreimbursable health care before they become eligible for Medicaid. In fact, over 47 percent of nursing home costs in the United States are paid by Medicaid for patients who were not initially poor (U.S. Congress, 1977). Medicaid expenditures are largely for institutional care, in part because it is costly, but also because many of the impoverished, disabled elderly have nowhere else to go after their resources are depleted. Nursing home care in the United States, unlike hospital care or nursing home care in most European countries, is a profit-making enterprise (Kane and Kane, 1978) and one supported primarily by public funds that pay for the care of the aged. There is little likelihood that this structure and orientation will change in the near future. Despite their importance, home health services represent less than 2 percent of Medicaid long-term care expenditures. Services vary widely from state to state and from community to community. In order to expand existing services and develop new home health services, the U.S. Public Health Service has a modest grant-in-aid program ($3 million in fiscal year 1977). In 1977, fifty-six projects were funded, forty-two of which were awarded for expansion of existing programs and fourteen for development of new services.

Despite the rapid increase in the costs of care provided in nursing homes, the quality of care in many of these institutions leaves much to be desired (Mendelson, 1975). From descriptions in reports and congressional hearings, one can only wonder how and why such care is tolerated in a society and by a medical profession that prides itself on excellence of care. In a recent report by the AFL-CIO, cited by the Senate Special Committee on Aging, abuses ranged from deaths due to negligence or injury to bribes, profiteering, unsanitary conditions, poor food, and violation of health and safety codes (U.S. Senate, 1978b). Thus, not only are the aged victims of the rapid price inflation in medical care services, reductions in state Medicaid programs, and declining benefits from the Medicare program, but programs for them are plagued by fraud and abuse by service providers, as well as by fraud and deception in the sale of private health insurance that is supposed to benefit the aged but often does just the opposite. Representative Claude Pepper, whose committee identified these abuses, described this as a $1-billion "ripoff" that constitutes "a full-scale national scandal" (*San Francisco Chronicle,* 1978c, p. 56).

Prior to the enactment of Medicare and Medicaid, public payments accounted for about 25 percent of national health expenditures. In 1976, public expenditures accounted for over 42 percent of all health expenses. For the elderly, after Medicare co-payments and premiums are deducted, Medicare paid for only 38 percent of their health care costs (U.S. Senate, 1978b). Medicare has done a great deal to meet the cost of illness among the aged who require short-term hospital care. Medicare Hospital Insurance (Part A) pays almost all of inpatient care through the first sixty days, with a modest deductible ($144 at current rates). What is needed is an extension of Medicare coverage for hospitalization beyond sixty days without the present limitations or coinsurance ($36 per day in 1978) for each day of care. Full protection against hospital costs without cost sharing, except for the initial deductible as under present law, could be provided at modest cost. The Supplementary Medical Insurance (Part B) is much less satisfactory. The aged person must pay a monthly premium, plus an annual deductible ($60 in 1977) if any medical bills are incurred, and 20

percent coinsurance for all "reasonable charges." Because of the
increasing number of physicians who are billing patients directly,
at charges well above those that Medicare considers "reasonable,"
the elderly are forced to pay more and more out of pocket as physician fees increase. Many of these problems could be solved by
combining Parts A and B of Medicare, eliminating the need for
the monthly premium paid by the beneficiary.

The two important gaps in Medicare's scope of coverage are
outpatient prescription drugs and long-term care. The elderly account for one quarter of all out-of-hospital drug expenditures. In
1976 they paid $2.78 billion for prescription drugs, 86 percent of
which was paid out of pocket. Coverage of outpatient prescription
drugs could be limited to those with costs over $150 annually (using
a deductible) or to those requiring specific drugs (for example,
antihypertensive drugs) for long-term use. The second major limitation of Medicare benefits relates to long-term care, including
home health services and nursing home care. Because of the high
cost of institutional care, many elderly are impoverished by these
expenses and thus become eligible for Medicaid coverage. What
is needed, however, is not just an extension of Medicare to cover
some long-term care costs, but available and effective support services designed to keep people out of institutions. For those who
require nursing home care, costs should be covered, but the system
should not be as heavily biased toward institutional care as it is
today.

Mental Health and Mental Health Services. Mental illness is a
serious problem for the aged. Although only 1 percent of persons
sixty-five and over are hospitalized in private or public mental institutions, it has been estimated that perhaps one half of the aged
in nursing homes, homes for the aged, and geriatric or chronic
disease hospitals suffer from significant psychiatric disorders (Busse
and Pfeiffer, 1977). The aged are confined to mental institutions
because of both psychiatric disorders and organic brain disease.
Although senile dementia is the most common of the organic brain
diseases, it often has its clinical expression in social circumstances
in which the aged individual has limited or no social contact or
social support system. The psychiatric disorders that may result in
long-term institutional care are primarily psychoses, such as schizo-

phrenia, that have caused the individual to be hospitalized for years.

The extent of mental illness among the elderly is difficult to define. Hospital, ambulatory care, and community studies provide quite different pictures of the problem. Although the aged make up 30 percent of patients in public mental hospitals and 11 percent of patients in private mental hospitals, they account for only 2 percent of patients seen in psychiatric clinics. The number of aged receiving care from private psychiatrists is also very small. In a number of community surveys, the percent of the aged with moderate to severe psychiatric problems ranged from 5 to 22 percent (Busse and Pfeiffer, 1977). It would seem that a great many aged do not receive needed psychiatric or mental health services. The fact that few old people seek or are provided psychiatric treatment on an ambulatory basis is often blamed on the elderly themselves. In reality, psychiatrists are poorly trained for this responsibility, health insurance (including Medicare) provides limited benefits, and there appears to be serious discrimination against the aged, at least in community mental health centers (U.S. Commission on Civil Rights, 1977).

Psychiatric and other mental health services may be provided in a variety of settings—private psychiatrists' or psychologists' offices, community mental health centers, hospital outpatient clinics and emergency rooms, neighborhood health centers, and ambulatory drug abuse and alcoholism centers. Short-term inpatient hospital care may be rendered in a community hospital or a psychiatric hospital, while long-term institutional care has traditionally taken place in state mental hospitals or veterans' hospitals. In recent years, more and more patients have been discharged into community settings only to end up in nursing homes. The U.S. Senate Special Committee on Aging has expressed particular concern about this: "The increasing numbers of older Americans discharged from mental hospitals into communities without resources to meet their needs was documented by the Committee on Aging during hearings in 1975. The committee reported then that the number of inpatients of all ages in state mental hospitals had dropped 44 percent between 1969 and 1974 (from 427,799 to 237,692). The number of elderly inpatients had decreased even more sharply, dropping 56 percent from 1969 to 1974 (from 135,322 to 59,685). Screening procedures to determine the best candidates for release were nonexistent in many states, and many elderly released to community care found themselves without attention and without help, including those placed in substandard boarding and nursing homes without access to mental health services" (U.S. Senate, 1978b, p. 76). The Senate committee also found that many patients who did not require continual institutional care could not be discharged because of the lack of adequate community mental health services.

Reliable data on expenditures for mental health services are lacking, but it has been estimated by the Department of Health, Education, and Welfare that:

- In 1976, $1.6 billion was spent for private outpatient psychiatric treatment, $1.5 billion for outpatient clinic services, and $1 billion for acute, short-term psychiatric hospitalization in general hospitals.
- For the same year, 1976, $4 billion was spent for longer-term care in public mental hospitals, $0.5 billion in private mental hospitals, and $1.1 billion for halfway houses, partial hospitalization, and other daycare settings (U.S. Department of Health, Education, and Welfare, 1977, p. 23).

Health insurance coverage for mental illness is quite limited. Although 68 percent of private health insurance plans provide some coverage for psychiatric hospitalization, in 32 percent such benefits are more limited than for physical illness and almost all place restrictions on psychiatric outpatient services. Medicare limits psychiatric care to 190 days and limits payments for outpatient care to a maximum of $250 per person. Medicaid coverage and reimbursement vary from state to state but in general are quite limited, particularly for the elderly (U.S. Department of Health, Education and Welfare, 1977).

Veterans' Medical Care. In addition to the expenditures for Medicare and Medicaid, the largest federal program of health services is that operated by the Veterans Administration (VA) for veterans with service-connected disabilities and those with nonservice-connected disabilities who cannot afford other care. In fiscal year 1977, VA programs spent $4.4 billion for the medical care of all veterans. An increasing share of VA expenditures will be for the care of elderly veterans. As the veteran populations from the Second World War and the Korean War age, there will be a very large increase in the number of elderly eligible for care in veterans' hospitals. In 1977, there were 2.37 million veterans sixty-five and over. This number is expected to double by 1982 and will increase even more rapidly after that. Surviving veterans from among the 4.4 million veterans age fifty-five to fifty-nine will enter the sixty-five-and-over group during the years 1983 to 1987 (Veterans Administration, 1977).

Approximately 16 percent of the applicants for VA hospital care are aged sixty-five and older, while 24 percent of all inpatients are in that same age group. Among psychiatric patients, approximately 25 percent are aged sixty-five and older (Veterans Administration, 1977). The percentage of long-term care services provided to the aged will undoubtedly rise, but data on this are not readily available. There are currently 75,000 veterans in "homes for the aged," with 26.3 percent in VA facilities or in those on contract to the VA (National Academy of Sciences, 1977). The needs of this increasing number of aged veterans have been identified by the National Research Council: "The VA clearly has two major groups of patients to whom it is providing service: a group of perhaps three million who use it occasionally for hospital care, and a much smaller group who reside in a VA hospital, nursing home, psychiatric, or domiciliary care facility. The latter group accounts for almost half the total VA inpatient census. The aging of the veteran population will increase the requirements for both acute and long-term care in the next ten to twenty years" (National Academy of Sciences, 1977, p. 33).

Other Health Services. The federal government supports a wide range of personal and community health services of possible benefit to the elderly. The U.S. Public Health Service provides grants to states for a variety of categorical health services, most of which are meant to aid children or young adults (for example, crippled children's services, family planning, and venereal disease control). The U.S. Public Health Service Hospitals, the Indian Health

Program, emergency medical services, migrant health services, home health services, and neighborhood or community health centers are some of the wide variety of federally funded health services for which the aged are eligible. But there is little information available on how many elderly actually benefit from these programs or what the outcomes have been. Surely some of the programs, such as home health services, are designed to meet the needs of the elderly requiring long-term care, but the few million dollars that the U.S. Public Health Service currently spends on home health services are just drops in the bucket, when the needs are examined. Age discrimination may be a factor in the failure of some of these programs to reach the aged. The U.S. Commission on Civil Rights found in its study of age discrimination that community health centers were neither accessible to the elderly nor responsive to their needs (U.S. Commission on Civil Rights, 1977).

During the past decade the federal government has initiated three separate, and as yet unrelated, programs designed to regulate the development of health care resources and the appropriateness of medical care and to improve the organization of services. The National Health Planning and Resource Development Act of 1974 (Public Law 93–641) created a mechanism to plan, develop, and regulate the supply of health care resources in local communities. The program established State Health Planning and Development Agencies (SHPDAs) and local Health Systems Agencies (HSAs) in every state. There are over 200 HSAs in various stages of development, which are primarily nonprofit private agencies responsible for developing health care plans for their areas and reviewing the need for new or additional hospital facilities. After three years of discussion and debate, national guidelines have been issued for widespread consideration and application. Many of the problems that have plagued area agencies on aging and state units on aging appear to be present in the HSAs and SHPDAs as well, but it is clearly too early to evaluate the effectiveness of the effort.

Professional Standards Review Organizations (PSROs) were established by Congress in the 1972 amendments to Title XVIII (Medicare) of the Social Security Act. The purpose of PSROs is to review the quality and appropriateness of hospital care provided Medicare and Medicaid patients. The need for the hospital admission, as well as the length of stay and the services provided, is examined. In 1978, PSROs were functioning in 154 of 195 designated areas, and in 1979 they are expected to review more than 60 percent of the Medicare and Medicaid hospital admissions. The aged might derive substantial benefit from the effective functioning of PSROs—particularly through reduction of unnecessary hospital admissions, surgical procedures, and laboratory tests. Controversy and conflict have surrounded the initiation of the PSRO program and, to date, the results of the efforts cannot be evaluated on a national basis. The third federal initiative designed to improve the delivery of health care and provide greater options for consumers is the Health Maintenance Organization (HMO) program, which was enacted in 1973 and amended in 1976. The early phases of this effort to develop hundreds of functioning prepaid group practice organizations have been hamstrung by insufficient funds, little technical expertise in Health, Education, and Welfare, red tape, and a lack of financial incentives in the Medicare and Medicaid programs. Although many new HMOs are developing without government assistance, the aged may not benefit initially from this development because many of these programs provide prepaid care to groups of employees.

Social Services. The House Select Committee on Aging (U.S. House, 1977a) has identified a range of social service programs for the elderly. They include: education programs for non-English-speaking elderly, legal services, multipurpose senior centers (Older Americans Act), a nutrition program for the elderly, services for low-income persons and public assistance recipients (Title XX of the Social Security Act), and state and community programs (Older Americans Act, Title III). Title XX of the Social Security Act is the major funding source for social services for all age groups. Federal funds are provided to the states, which have wide flexibility in determining who will be eligible and what services will be provided. A number of services are potentially useful to the aged. However, after only two years of program operation, it has not been possible to identify the numbers of elderly served or the services they have received. During the quarter ending June 30, 1976, $117.2 million, or 17.5 percent of the Title XX (social services) expenditures, were spent for chore services, adult daycare, home-delivered or aggregate meals, homemaker services, and home management services that might be of most direct benefit to the aged.

The U.S. Commission on Civil Rights, in its age discrimination study, found a variety of legislative actions and administrative decisions at the state level that discriminated against the aged in the allocation of Title XX funds and services. For example, administrators have concentrated services on recipients of Aid to Families with Dependent Children (AFDC) so that they may become employed. The basis for this was a narrow interpretation of the Title XX objectives; that is, assisting individuals to maintain self-sufficiency in order to achieve economic self-support (U.S. Commission on Civil Rights, 1977, p. 32). In a number of states, legislators have enacted age-specific legislation (for example, child abuse laws) without providing funds to implement the programs. As a result, most of the available Title XX funds must be used for these categorical problems, and little is left to serve the needs of the aged. Prior commitment of funds, usually for services to children and families, coupled with the federal funding limits, has been an additional factor limiting social services for the aged.

What evidence is available suggests that the needs of the elderly receive scant attention in federally supported rehabilitation and education programs. The U.S. Commission on Civil Rights examined a number of federally supported programs, including legal services, Basic Vocational Rehabilitation, State Vocational Education, and Adult Basic Education. In each program, the commission found evidence of discrimination on the basis of age. In some programs, such as vocational rehabilitation, the discrimination against the aged was marked, while in others the problems were less severe (U.S. Commission on Civil Rights, 1977). It is estimated that of the disabled persons rehabilitated through the state-federal program of Vocational Rehabilitation, approximately two percent are over sixty-five (U.S. Department of Health, Education, and Welfare, 1978). The commission's report included nineteen findings of discrimination and twelve recommendations for legislative changes and administrative actions to deal with the problem. The recommendations focused particularly on the need for changes in the Age Discrimination Act and the need for forceful enforcement of its current provisions (U.S. Commission on Civil Rights, 1977, pp. 10–77, 82–103).

Transportation

Although public transportation is a vital service for millions of the elderly who do not own their own automobiles (38 percent of older households), there has been little national attention devoted to the many problems involved. In some communities the elderly are able to ride municipal buses, railways, or subways for reduced fares. In many cases, however, the physical barriers to access to public transportation preclude their use. There are many local volunteer organizations that provide van or automobile transportation for the handicapped and the elderly. In some communities, the elderly are reimbursed by the local government for the cost of taxi fare to needed medical or dental care. Senior centers may also provide transportation for center activities to the elderly who might not otherwise be able to participate.

The Administration on Aging provides funds, through area agencies on aging, to pay for local transportation for the elderly, which was given a high priority by Congress as a linking or access service. However, the Department of Transportation apparently has not considered the transportation needs of the elderly a high priority. Four programs administered by the Transportation department are related to the elderly: Capital Assistance grants for use by public agencies, Capital Assistance grants for use by private nonprofit groups, reduced fares, and capital and operating assistance grants that may benefit the elderly. For the capital grant programs only 2 percent of the funds must be set aside for equipment or services designed to meet the needs of the elderly or the handicapped. More effective in providing the elderly with access to needed public transportation has been the requirement in the Urban Mass Transportation Act that mass transportation companies receiving federal funds for either capital or operating expenses must charge elderly and handicapped individuals no more than half fare, except during peak hours.

Training and Research Programs

Although training and research programs are considered among the major programs benefiting the elderly by the House Select Committee on Aging, and at least a half dozen such programs can be found in the *1978 Catalog of Federal Domestic Assistance,* we have excluded these programs from this analysis because they do not provide services directly to the elderly.

Eighty Programs Later

What does it all add up to? More than eighty federal programs designed to benefit the elderly directly or indirectly and over $120 billion in federal expenditures annually should produce significant results. The results too often are not significant, however, and certainly the programs do not meet the goals defined in the Older Americans Act. Indeed, most do not meet their own often ambitious and ambiguous goals. The end result is that the status of the aged, relative to other age groups, has been altered very little by these federal programs. There has been little or no change in power relationships, the allocation of resources, or the dominance of public policy decisions by special interests. Of course, without some of the programs, particularly Social Security and Medicare, the status of the aged in the United States would be even more dismal than it is today.

We have found it difficult and frustrating to attempt to evaluate the outcomes of these many federal programs. It is appalling how little information is really available to assist policy makers in judgments about the outcome and effectiveness of programs. This lack of accountability makes it impossible to determine what really works. Even when programs are effective, it is often difficult to determine why and thus impossible to replicate successes on a broad scale. The current federal programs designed to assist the elderly range from income support to research training, from volunteer services to public housing, from transportation subsidies to Medicare. In the 1960s there were strong federal leadership and multiple federal initiatives to deal with the major domestic social problems of the nation, including the problems of the aged. In the 1970s, as Social Security payments rose, Medicare and food stamp expenditures increased, and other programs grew without resolving the problems, new approaches were called for. New federalism and revenue sharing emerged as major policy developments. As new programs were added to the old, growing concern was expressed about the multiplicity of programs and the difficulties encountered by the elderly attempting to find their way through the maze. Planning and coordination were offered as answers to the "chaotic fragmentation in federal programs serving the elderly" (U.S. House, 1977b, app. p. 139). The Older Americans Act was viewed as a potential vehicle to apply the policies of revenue sharing and new federalism to the aged, and it was to be the basis for the planning and smooth coordination of services. We turn next to an examination of how this strategy was put into effect.

Carroll L. Estes
Lenore Gerard

VI

Achievements
and Problems of
the Older Americans Act

There is no doubt that the programs of the Older Americans Act directly help many older persons. . . . Unfortunately, these positive features of the Older Americans Act go hand in hand with a series of weaknesses, [among them, that] the extensive range of programmatic responsibilities has been elaborated without much sense of priority . . . [and that] the programmatic agenda and the bureaucratic network have been developed with sufficient fanfare to create a cruel illusion that a variety of problems can eventually be solved through funding and implementation under the Older Americans Act [Binstock, 1978, p. 1838].

Although the Older Americans Act was initially designed to stimulate the development of needed services for the elderly, it became increasingly evident as the years passed that there was a need to provide a better means for planning and coordinating the programs serving the elderly. Congress used the Older Americans Act to plan and coordinate and created the area agencies on aging for this purpose in 1973. Recently Congress has insisted that the Administration on Aging play a stronger coordinating role within the federal government.

Major obstacles make it virtually impossible for the Administration on Aging to achieve the congressional goals of both planning and coordination. For example, there is no national social policy for the elderly, federal programs are organized on functional rather than clientele lines, and the agency lacks authority even within the Department of Health, Education, and Welfare to coordinate major programs in health and social services, let alone those in other departments and agencies.

Merely coordinating the eighty federal programs providing or financing services that might be utilized by the elderly would involve at least twenty-three different federal agencies in seventeen departments or independent agencies with separate authorizations and appropriations. During fiscal year 1976 the Administration on Aging succeeded in negotiating and signing twenty formal working agreements with other federal departments and agencies that cut across all aspects of health, income, housing, education, and transportation (Administration on Aging, 1978, p. 30). However, one major problem with these interagency/intraagency agreements is their wide variability and lack of authority; many are simply agreements to agree. Too often these agreements have achieved little or nothing toward actually improving the coordination of services to the elderly (U.S. General Accounting Office, 1977a, p. 54).

Federal and federal-state joint programs are the major source of funding for services for the elderly (Westat, 1978b, p. V:11). Definitions, eligibility criteria, and regulations governing utilization, administration, and authority reside at either the federal or state level, depending on how the programs are financed. All these programs have an important influence on planning and coordination efforts at the local level. But the crucial role of area agencies within these state-federal programs, especially Medicare, Medicaid, and Title XX, remains unclear and unspecified in the Older Americans Act. The dilemma surrounding the area agencies' mandate to "coordinate" local programs and services, which remain fragmented at the federal level, has been repeatedly stressed in agency and congressional reports.

The central dilemmas and solutions concerning fragmentation of services and programs for the elderly were explored by the House Select Committee on Aging (U.S. House, 1977a). Wit-

nesses saw fragmentation as resulting from: (1) insufficient resources at the local level to provide services, (2) insufficient dollars
for the development of expertise and management technology,
(3) ambiguity and conflict over jurisdictional authority at the federal, state, and local levels, and (4) lack of a comprehensive federal
social policy. Roemer, Frink, and Kramer have observed that fragmentation of health and social services emanating from the pluralistic character of government will not "be modified by consolidation or coordination of agencies alone" (1975, p. 4) and that the
salient characteristic of fragmentation is the "lack of an integrated
policy and purpose by government to link the many parts of the
system" (p. 15). Though many analysts have emphasized the need
for a larger federal role and commitment for effective planning
and coordination, ambiguity surrounding area agencies as a focal
point for programs of the elderly is structurally embedded in the
new federalism strategy. In addition, the lack of specification of
what coordination is or of how to go about achieving it is also a
problem inherent in the new federalism strategy, which provides
local level agencies with the discretion to answer these questions
for themselves.

   Johnson has observed that although the more than five
hundred area agencies on aging were established with laudable intent, "many if not most of them are dysfunctional" (U.S. House,
1977e, p. 151). Some analysts claim that the basic problems of area
agencies stem from insufficient resources to realize objectives
(Howenstine, Miller, and Tucker, 1975; U.S. House, 1977e), while
others emphasize that the problems are associated with three potentially conflicting roles—planning, service delivery, and advocacy. If area agencies on aging "seem to be overwhelmed by demands that have little to do with everyday needs of the elderly,"
as some members of Congress observed (U.S. Senate, 1976a,
pp. 15–16), it is because they spend most of their time trying to
fulfill their basic responsibilities as planning and coordinating bodies. Support for the idea of area agencies as planning and coordinating units with strictly limited roles in direct provision of service has not wavered and, in fact, the 1978 Older Americans Act
reauthorization testimony strengthened this basic concept.

   There is, however, a clear lack of specificity concerning what
coordination is, how the direct service and supportive service net-

works are to work, and what their interorganizational structures and processes can or should be (Howenstine, Miller, and Tucker, 1975). As one congressional witness noted: "There is no operating definition of coordination in [Administration on Aging] regulations. There is a rather broad definition of a coordinated, comprehensive service delivery system, and several requirements to coordinate, but nothing that tells the aging network what [the administration] means by coordination and what steps can be taken to reach that goal. It's as if the federal level is saying to the state and local levels, 'you must coordinate—but coordination is anything you want it to be' " (Cutler in U.S. House, 1977e, p. 115). Repeated testimony from agencies in the aging network has emphasized the need for local discretion, arguing that the problem is that the area agencies do not have the skill or the time to conceptualize what effective coordination is.

Commenting on the problems of fragmentation and lack of coordination, Maggie Kuhn, national convenor of the Gray Panthers, expressed views shared by many elderly:

> There is further fragmentation and duplication of services because the state and area offices on aging have been placed without proper regard for the programs already in operation by established social agencies and denominational groups; coordinated planning and budgeting are done with the traditional agencies for information and referral services, counseling services, meals on wheels, health screening, and so forth. Private agencies operate these programs with the help of many volunteers and private contributions. However, we have observed few efforts to bring nongovernmental, private agency services and governmental services together. In metropolitan areas like New York City and Chicago, we have seen that the area offices operate on a highly centralized basis and are administered by American management techniques. Departments of aging are rapidly becoming bureaucracies, with their staffs hobnobbing with other staffs and further and further removed from daily contact with the people to be served—all this with limited input from the ideas and experiences of the older person [Kuhn in U.S. House, 1977a].

Gerontological experts and consultants have emphasized the viability of a comprehensive planning process at the national, state, and local levels and have seen it as the solution to the problem of fragmentation of services: "[T]he services that older persons need are provided by a complex of public and private agencies . . . rarely does a provider . . . attempt to assess an older person's needs on a comprehensive basis. Consequently, an older person . . . seeks out the combination of agencies that can meet [his needs]. . . . much of this can be changed. Those states, area agencies, and local aging organizations which have organized interagency planning processes are the ones which have been most successful in treating the older person as a whole person. . . . we should be able to pull together many of the myriad public and private agencies . . . to meet the multiple needs of our older Americans. To be successful at the area and local level, comprehensive planning must first be carefully designed and supported at the national and state levels" (Newton in U.S. House, 1977a, p. 106).

The 1978 amendments to the Older Americans Act have consolidated programs of former Titles III, V, and VII (area planning, senior centers, and nutrition) into one Title III with authorizations remaining separate for each program; model projects are now part of Title IV (research and training), and the employment program (formerly Title IX) is now called Title V. The 1978 amendments did not, however, change the emphasis on the indirect services of planning, pooling, and coordination, the latter two of which are identified in the Older Americans Act as "social service" activities and are accounted for under funds for services (not administration). The assumption is that "there is an opportunity for implementing these provisions in all planning and service areas and . . . then . . . some older persons [will] receive services that they otherwise would not receive. This is why . . . Congress placed major emphasis . . . on the coordination of services" (U.S. House, 1975, p. 113).

Evaluating Area Agencies

The major Administration on Aging evaluation of area agencies and the primary data source on the activities and effectiveness of these agencies is the Westat study. The first Westat report, covering the period from July 1974 to June 1976, is based on interviews in thirty-nine area agencies in twenty-seven states. Sampled were 1283 service providers in the thirty-nine planning and service areas, staff in twenty-seven state units, thirty-seven advisory council members, and nineteen umbrella agency representatives. The Westat (1978a, p. xvii) study assessed the effectiveness of area agencies from several perspectives by examining:

1. The change in the characteristics of the services delivered to the elderly and the types of services available
2. Improvements in services attributable, in part at least, to area agency endeavors
3. The percent of area agency attempts to improve services that succeeded
4. The extent to which area agencies contributed to the attainment of the following objective: the development of more comprehensive, coordinated delivery systems concerned with the needs of the elderly

Seventy-two percent of area agency directors (out of a sample of thirty-nine) reported the official purpose of an agency to be planning, with only 15 percent of agency directors reporting advocacy as the official purpose. The area agency's primary purpose was reported by these same directors as planning (43 percent), coordination (41 percent), and advocacy (31 percent). A mere 13 percent of agency directors reported that their primary purpose was to enable the elderly to remain at home and/or to improve conditions of the elderly, and a negligible 3 percent of directors reported that their agency's primary purpose was to provide the elderly with needed services (Westat, 1978a, p. IV:5).

Westat reported that the primary activities of area agencies were general program development and coordination. Program development and coordination comprised an average of 27 percent and 19 percent of all area agency activities, respectively. Further, it was found that the coordination, pooling, and training and technical assistance activities performed most frequently by area agencies accounted for more than half of all reported agency activities in some planning and service areas (Westat, 1978a, p. V:7).

The Westat evaluation of agency effectiveness in the development of more comprehensive, coordinated service delivery systems employed three kinds of measures:

First, *measures of system comprehensiveness* covered volume of services, staff time spent in direct service provision, accessibility of services, area served, fees paid by the elderly, eligibility requirements, and outreach activities. One of the major findings of the Westat study was an overall improvement in service delivery to the elderly; thus, 93 percent of all service providers showed an improvement in at least one of the seventeen service characteristics. The highest rates of improvement associated with system comprehensiveness were in the volume of services; the least improvement was found in accessibility of services. The range of services increased during the summer of 1974 to the summer of 1976, with information and referral ranking first and counseling second. These findings are rather puzzling since the area agency emphasis is on improving access of the elderly to services, yet Westat reported that accessibility of services showed the lowest rate of improvement. Of the operational components to the improvement of access—geographic accessibility, economic accessibility, and awareness of services available—the contribution of the area agencies was in increased activities in information and referral and outreach programs.

Second, *measures of system coordination* covered efforts to coordinate services, contracts with local officials, senior citizens, and other groups, involvement of elderly in planning and priority setting, and information and referral activities. While system coordination showed the highest improvement in program objectives during the period from 1974 to 1976, there are significant qualifications to these coordination achievements. As analyzed and reported, the data are undifferentiated, limited primarily to service changes/improvements with emphasis on the subcontracted providers of area agencies and a sample of other providers within the aging network. Thus it is impossible to differentiate among improvement rates of the various agencies and activities linked to area agencies. In addition, there is no basis for determining whether the changes relate to the "needs" of the people or the "needs" of the agency. The Westat study does not measure the impact of area agency efforts at coordination upon the elderly or include the views and experiences of the beneficiaries, nor does Westat analyze the structural problems of coordination. Area agencies have no control over the most crucial aspects pertaining to coordination—for example, accessibility to the distribution of resources of major federal and federal-state programs such as Medicare and Medicaid. While it appears that area agencies can best achieve coordination in the "system" through information and referral services and through interaction within the aging network, these are minimal steps that do not address the structural problems of coordination in the broader system.

Limitations in the findings on coordination also inhere in the ambiguity and breadth of the concept and its measurement. The Westat study identified as operational components of system coordination: "(1) degree of interaction of actors in the system; (2) involvement of other organizations and individuals; (3) cross referring clients; (4) degree of joint efforts in service delivery; and, (5) the extent of services matching needs" (Westat, 1978a, p. II:10). While these coordination measures reflect activity-interaction rates (for example, contacts and efforts to coordinate), such measures are typically called input measures or measures of effort. They do not, however, provide us with any substantive data pertaining to outcome in terms of actual improvements in community-wide coordination of services. The area where one would expect to see some measurable benefits of area agency coordination efforts—increase in budget allocations and/or services for the elderly—is discussed under "system concern," and even there its continued emphasis upon coordination and planning leaves room for considerable skepticism about its actual achievements.

Difficulties in operationalizing the concept of coordination are not unique to Westat researchers. Marmor and Kutza (1975) identified multiple conceptions of the meaning of the terms *comprehensiveness* and *coordination* and reported six different problems under the general rubric of coordination issues, each of which calls for a different policy-intervention strategy: (1) fragmentation, (2) duplication of service, (3) gaps in services, (4) inaccessibility of services, (5) discontinuity of serial and sequential service interventions, and (6) incoherency among simultaneous interventions. Although there is no consensus as to what coordination means, one commonality is that it is always considered from the point of view of the service providers rather than the service beneficiaries.

O'Brien and Wetle (1975) noted similar conceptual problems, and in a study of more than three hundred area agency on aging directors, Tobin, Davidson, and Sack (1976) found that 45 to 52 percent of agency directors regarded the following terms as "very" or "somewhat ambiguous": (1) effectiveness, (2) linkage of services, (3) pooling untapped resources, (4) comprehensiveness, and (5) coordinated services. Such conceptual fuzziness obviously creates measurement problems for the researcher; but, more significantly, it fosters lack of accountability in implementation of the program. As discussed throughout this book, a basic shortcoming of the Older Americans Act is its lack of specificity concerning what coordination is, how the comprehensive delivery system is supposed to work, and what the interorganizational structures and processes should be. Its broad mandate provides the flexibility and discretion at the local level that are keystones of the new federalism, and these policies are widely supported by the national organizations spawned by the Older Americans Act. But this same mandate makes it difficult to hold local agencies accountable for their policies.

Third, *measures of system concern for the elderly* included percent of elderly clients, percent of budget used, budget requests, percent of low-income or minority elderly, training, and activity to determine impact of services. *System concern for the elderly* received the lowest improvement rate. Less than half the service providers reported an improvement on any of the measures; an improvement rate of less than 45 percent on each of the measures was experienced by half the planning and service areas of the area agencies studied. Significantly, this is the one area to include fiscal data of service providers that indicated progress. Disappointing, however, is the fact that an unknown number of these alleged improvements merely reflect standing in place in a rising resource market. Changes pertaining to providers' expenditures on services for the elderly were attributed principally to an increase in the availability of funds for services, with the elderly's share remaining unchanged (Westat, 1978a). Furthermore, although two thirds of the providers reported a budget increase for the elderly between 1974 and 1976, there are major qualifications to this "progress." The majority of service providers who increased expenditures for the elderly did so by less than 5 percent; and those who increased expenditures still spent less in services for the elderly than did providers who decreased or held expenditures constant (Westat, 1978a).

The Administration on Aging has reported optimistically on the pooling success of its Title III program. The $122 million in Title III appropriations in fiscal year 1977 were instrumental in tapping existing resources and pooling more than $400 million, about half cash and half in-kind resources. Seventy percent of these dollars were federal funds, 20 percent were local, and 10 percent were state funds. The major categories of pooled resources were (1) Title XX (Social Security Act), (2) Medicaid, (3) Comprehensive Training and Employment Act, and (4) Housing and Urban Development programs (excluding community development). These "pooled" funds illustrate the difficulty of defining what pooling is. Medicaid funds, for example, are paid to providers when eligible low-income elderly use covered services. Food stamps also represent expenditures on behalf of eligible individuals. How and to what extent the area agencies assisted individuals in "pooling" Medicaid or food stamps is not clear. The largest allocation of funds, Title XX social services, represents a major potential for "pooling." Again, however, reports do not indicate what role the area agencies played in obtaining the services for the elderly. (Additional questions about the reliability and validity of the pooling data reported are discussed at length in Chapter Seven.)

Regrettably, advocacy was accorded little emphasis in the Westat evaluation. Its focus instead was on "those activities which were intended to bring about changes in services to the elderly offered by service providers in their planning and service area. Other activities, such as contract management and political advocacy, received much less attention" (Westat, 1978a, p. xix). The meager available data concerning the aged as advocates relate primarily to their functions on advisory committees in conjunction with state units or area agencies. The first such study, conducted prior to the 1973 amendments that created area agencies, reported on state unit committees in forty-nine states (Alaska was excluded) (Binstock, 1972b). The membership composition of these committees was heavily weighted toward technical and professional experts and agency and organization representatives—averaging 10.6 members per state unit committee, while there were 4.1 older Americans per committee (with a total committee size averaging about 15). Binstock's research found that these committees primarily responded to, rather than initiated, proposals, and it described them in a large majority of the cases as entirely void of major controversy. Binstock reported that the state unit committees functioned most importantly as sources of political strength, as liaison vehicles, and as sounding boards. But only eight of the forty-nine state units reported policy making among the functions of these committees. Binstock's study also revealed that the state units with a larger proportion of consumers on their advisory and policy-making committees showed an increased orientation toward development of regional and local advocacy groups. In contrast, representation of the voluntary sector on the committee reinforced efforts to involve that sector.

Another study of state unit advisory committees conducted by Applied Management Sciences (1975) three years later found the same sounding-board and political liaison roles. The state units used advisory committees chiefly to combat difficulties due to a state's particular legislative mechanisms or political constraints on active political partisanship by state agencies. An additional factor reported as contributory to the effective functioning of state unit advisory committees was the selection of members skilled in areas pertinent to committee functions—for example, geriatric specialists and public agency administrators—versus membership selection mainly based on strict socioeconomic and demographic characteristics. As a result, advisory committees often have few elderly members, particularly from low-income and minority groups.

Another 1975 study of advocacy in the field of aging found that state units on aging kept a lower profile than area agencies in advocacy for vulnerable groups such as the elderly poor, ethnic minorities, and those living in rural areas. For all agencies, interaction with these groups was "spotty and undeveloped" (Human

Resources Corporation, 1975, p. 126). A more recent study of the participation of 100 advisory council members in area agencies reveals that the most active members were engaged in follow-up activities: "visiting sites to monitor programs; reviewing grant applications; preparing reports; investigating complaints [of] program participants; testifying at hearings . . . speaking out as consumer advocates at other public meetings; and lobbying" (Fleisher and Kaplan, 1978, p. 1). The study also noted that "these councils . . . do not meet the [older persons'] expectations [for] personal involvement. Attention [needs to be given to] more responsive structures so that the expertise of consumer members is utilized to the fullest. Staff needs to guard against underestimating . . . capabilities of consumer members" (p. 5).

Westat found that advocacy accounted for a small proportion of area agency effort in each of the three broad program objectives: system comprehensiveness (6 percent); system coordination (19 percent); and system concern for the elderly (5 percent) (1978a, p. III:22). Other relevant Westat findings are that advisory council representatives consider themselves most useful to the area agency in representing the elderly in policy-making situations, and least useful in organizing groups of elderly persons for planning and priority-setting input. Also, two fifths of the advisory councils had taken actions during the evaluation period to improve services to the elderly through agents other than the area agencies. Eighty-eight percent of the councils Westat studied had attempted to influence the legislative process for the benefit of the elderly; 75 percent had disseminated information to the community about the needs of the elderly; and 50 percent had organized new groups of older Americans (Westat, 1978a, pp. VII:18–19).

A recent survey of 555 area agencies conducted by the House Select Committee on Aging shows that 89 percent of these agencies believed that advocacy could potentially improve the welfare of the aged in their areas (U.S. House, 1978e, p. 11). But their estimate that a total of $6.5 million and an average of 1.9 staff are needed for each area agency in order to meet these advocacy potentials is discouraging. These data generally substantiate Steinberg's earlier conclusions from a study of ninety-seven area agencies: "[Area agencies] reported difficulties with . . . participation of the elderly in advisory councils and in other mechanisms of consumer feedback" (1976, p. 30).

It is clear from these findings that advocacy activities play a lesser role in state unit and area agency efforts than most other responsibilities, although theoretically they are the key to the pooling of existing resources, development of new resources, and establishment of state units and area agencies as the focal points for state and local services for the aged. These findings, along with the analysis in Chapter Nine of the limited advocacy roles in national programs for the aged, indicate that pressure for major policy advances and resource commitments required for the nation's aged most likely will have to come from outside the structures of such existing federal programs as the Older Americans Act.

Having reviewed all components of the area planning strategy, what can we learn from available studies about policy design and implementation issues and choices? Recommendations by all categories of Westat respondents for improved area agency effectiveness focused first on funding and staffing. The second most important concern for area agencies was more flexibility and authority. In contrast, other types of respondents (state units, advisory committees, community leaders) uniformly gave second priority to increasing area agency attention to specific services, thus highlighting the tension between the emphasis on indirect services (planning, pooling, coordination) and on direct services in the Older Americans Act. Responses to a similar question concerning barriers to area agency effectiveness brought out, first, the perceived lack of sufficient resources; second, poor communication/coordination with other groups; and third, public apathy (Westat, 1978a, pp. IV:60–62).

The plea for more resources is nearly universal in most area agency studies (Steinberg, 1976; Tobin, Davidson, and Sack, 1976; Howenstine, Miller, and Tucker, 1975; Marmor and Kutza, 1975). Almost as frequently, pleas are recorded for more and/or better coordination in spite of the fact that much of the same literature is replete with discussions of the difficulty and barriers to coordination. The consistency and regularity of these expressions are instructive, for they signal the underlying acceptance of the planning/coordination strategy as appropriate and in need only of fine-tuning adjustments rather than as irrelevant and possibly even dangerous to the interests of the aged ill and poor.

The Services Package

The 1978 Older Americans Act Amendments illustrate congressional concern for dollar effectiveness and efficiency. Currently, each area agency is required to expend 50 percent of its allotment on supportive services associated with access—transportation, outreach, information and referral, and in-home and legal services. In addition to this controversial targeting of services, the 1978 amendments emphasized that area agency activities must be coordinated with the development of senior centers and nutrition services. Thus, Titles III, V, and VII are now consolidated into one Title III services package. A major proportion of area agencies (59.2 percent) reported that between 51 and 100 percent of their total budget was allocated to purchase of services (U.S. House, 1978e, p. 4), while less than 6 percent of their budgets was spent on provision of direct services. Although Westat's sample of area agencies did include those that provided services directly to the elderly, very little information on direct services was gathered because "direct services were severely limited by law" (Westat, 1978a, p. II:20). Thus, the bulk of the data reported by Westat pertains to the purchase of supporting and gap-filling services for the elderly.

According to Westat, the area agencies studied projected that an average of $82,000 would be expended on supporting services and $45,000 on gap-filling services for fiscal year 1976. For the 45 percent of the area agencies with Title VII (nutrition) expenditures, the average amount projected for nutritional services was $191,000. Although some agencies projected substantial expenditures for their services, about one quarter expected to spend $50 thousand or less on supporting services and 54 percent of the agencies planned to spend $50 thousand or less on gap-filling services. Eleven percent planned to spend nothing for support services and 3 percent planned no expenditures for gap-filling services (Westat, 1978b, pp. IV:19–20). Unfortunately, it is impossible to determine the proportion of the total area agency budgets allocated for such services because of Westat's budget reporting methods. Westat does indicate that the mean (average) area agency budget total from Title III funds in fiscal year 1976 was $188,000; for Title VII (for the area agencies administering nutrition projects), it was $115,000; and for other Administration on Aging funds, it was $5,000 (Westat, 1978b, p. IV:12, Table 4–9). Subsequent Westat tables appear to indicate there are other funding sources and amounts, but whether these are additional to the required "match" is not clear. Thus, there is no way to learn average or mean area agency budget size (the statistical measure that was used to describe projected social services expenditures), although the median area agency budget is reported at $310,000 (Westat, 1978b, p. IV:16). Regrettably, there are also no report data on the amount of funds allocated to the various services but only on the number and types of services. Perhaps the most important finding is that it is impossible to tell either relative input in resources area agencies are committing to social services or the impact of such service provision efforts on the aged. Certainly the data on absolute dollars that the area agencies anticipated they would expend on gap-filling and supporting services are discouraging—only about $127,000 per planning and service area was projected for 1976.

A pattern of emphasis on "linking and accessing" services has been relatively constant since the inception of area agencies, except for the added emphasis on priority services incorporated in the 1975 amendments to the Older Americans Act (transportation, home services, legal counseling, and residential repair and renovation) and reaffirmed in slightly modified form in the 1978 amendments.

In fiscal year 1977, the order of specified services expenditures was: first, transportation; second, in-home services; and third, information and referral. A new category for outreach ranked fourth. Expenditures for home repair services increased, slightly exceeding those for legal services for the first time, although both of them almost tied for fifth rank.

Senior Centers. Although created by the 1973 amendments to the Older Americans Act, no appropriation was made for senior centers until the transition quarter of fiscal year 1976 (June 30, 1976 to September 30, 1976). Until the 1978 amendments, Title V funds were provided only for the acquisition, renovation, or alteration of a facility that would serve as a multipurpose senior center. Initial funding supported alteration and renovation in 457 centers; 69 were given funds for equipment; and 23 facilities were acquired with the funds. In fiscal year 1977, the $20 million appropriated supported approximately 1,500 senior center facilities. Churches, schools, theaters, community centers, office buildings, stores, warehouses, hotels, motels, and even mobile homes were modified with Title V funds. In addition, in fiscal year 1978 it was possible for the first time for Title V funding to be employed for staff support. Later funding will make it possible to renovate or alter 2,340 multipurpose senior centers and acquire 260 facilities to be used as centers.

The services provided by multipurpose senior centers may extend beyond their traditional emphasis upon recreation. Although growth of the senior center movement has been slowed by an initial lack of funds (it first gained appropriations in 1976), Congress has recently lent support to the idea of senior centers as appropriate settings for a comprehensive single-entry service system. Older Americans Act amendments of 1978 give area agencies the discretion to designate senior centers as focal points for comprehensive services in their community. What this means or how it will be implemented, however, remains unclear. Meanwhile, senior center advocates continue to struggle against the popular conception of senior centers as largely recreational facilities rather than as centers for health and social services. In 1973 the term *multipurpose senior center* was defined in Title V of the Older Americans Act as a community facility for the organization and provision of a broad spectrum of services—health, social, and educational— as well as facilities for recreational activities for older persons. But this definition leaves considerable ambiguity as to the functions of senior centers. Title V provides no specific mandates concerning the organization or complement of social and health services to be provided; instead, senior center funding emphasized finance-related concepts—providing grants for their alteration, acquisition, and renovation; authorizing use of federal mortgage insurance to guarantee loans; reducing mortgage interest payments on loans; and authorizing grants to assist in staffing costs.

The 1978 reauthorization hearings witnessed overwhelming support for the inclusion of an additional provision for "limited new construction" in circumstances where no other suitable facility is available. Given increasing support for senior center expansion and anticipated rises in fiscal appropriations, the multipurpose senior center program may benefit the construction industry more than it does the elderly themselves. In fact, at a hearing before the House Committee on Appropriations in 1977, Title V was praised as generating increased economic activity: "Since most of the funds are spent for building supplies and salaries of workmen, it generates increased economic activity in addition to providing needed service facilities" (Martinez in U.S. House, 1977b, p. 789). This trend toward expansion of senior centers may continue to gain momentum, for it may be an expedient way to demonstrate that something tangible is being done for the aged.

Nutrition Programs for the Elderly. The largest appropriation for any program funded through the Older Americans Act is for nutrition. In 1977, Title VII encompassed more than 1,047 nutrition projects service meals at 9,166 congregate sites in every state. Meals were served daily in a variety of locations: religious facilities (24 percent), senior centers (22 percent), housing complexes (13 percent), schools (4 percent), restaurants (2 percent), and other facilities. More than 450,000 meals were served daily to an estimated 2,854,755 elderly people during the year, 67 percent of whom were low income and 22 percent minorities. Over 100,000 elderly volunteers and 27,000 younger volunteers assisted. Approximately 85 percent of the meals were served at congregate sites, and 15 percent were served to the homebound elderly. In addition to the $225 million spent by nutrition projects in fiscal year 1977, the Department of Agriculture provided $30 million in commodities to the nutrition projects. The commodities are issued on the basis of 27.25 cents per meal (the costs per meals were estimated to be $1.73, while the total program cost per meals was estimated by the Administration on Aging to be $2.46). In general, there is enthusiastic support for the nutrition program, largely because it is one of the few unambiguous direct services in the Older Americans Act and a program for which eligibility is automatic at age sixty, with none of the red tape characteristic of many other programs.

Nevertheless, several major areas of concern exist about the program, two of which the 1978 amendments to the Older Americans Act attempted to resolve. First, the amendments consolidated Titles III, V, and VII in the hope of abating a long and sometimes bitter power struggle between the area planning agencies and the formerly independent nutrition agencies (which between 1972 and 1978 were administered by the state unit on aging, unless the state unit chose to have its area agencies administer the program). Second, the amendments included Senator Edward Kennedy's legislation to provide for home-delivered meals to homebound older Americans, increasing available nutrition appropriations beyond the 20 percent maximum permitted under Title VII prior to 1978.

Other concerns, still unresolved, relate to the use of commodities, the effect of the program's universal eligibility requirements, and the level of assistance that this small program actually provides in relation to need. In 1977 the Senate Special Committee noted that "the commodities provision has been of great assistance . . . in increasing the number of meals served. However, complaints increased over . . . the cost of transporting and storing such commodities . . . and their value in the diet. Many . . . were foods which could not be chewed and digested by older persons. Some contained spices . . . discouraged in certain diets" (U.S. Senate, 1978b, p. 126).

Program eligibility is intrinsically linked with equity—should priorities be set for those in the greatest need or should universal criteria be adopted favoring those who already have access to public service programs? This issue is particularly important in the national meals program, not only because it is one of the few tangible services provided by the Older Americans Act but also because the waiting lists are almost double the number of daily meals currently served (Anderson in U.S. Senate, 1978a). These equity-related issues will probably assume greater importance because the nutrition program is likely to continue expanding as a result of its congressional popularity. These programs are additionally important insofar as they may become focal points for comprehensive services delivery.

Community Service Employment for Older Americans. This program is intended to assist low-income persons fifty-five and older by promoting useful part-time work opportunities in community service activities. Unlike other Older Americans Act programs, it is not administered by the Administration on Aging but through the Department of Labor. In fiscal year 1972 the program employed slightly over 5,000 older workers in service activities in hospitals, churches, parks, and schools "to give them a new sense of pride and purpose" (U.S. Senate, 1973b, p. 163). In fiscal year 1974, $10 million was appropriated to provide support for 3,300 part-time jobs. As described in Chapter Three, the Older American Community Service Employment Act was incorporated into the Older Americans Act in 1975. Although the program has expanded substantially in dollar terms and in the number of elderly employed as a result, this type of categorical approach fails to meet even a minimum goal for employment. When multiple billions of dollars are available for youth employment and training and less than one percent of that amount is available for employment of the elderly, it is evident why employers give youth a priority. Discrimination and forced retirement, as noted previously, further aggravate the problem. Equally noteworthy is the observation that, in the face of the gross insufficiency of this extremely small program (that can only be described as symbolic), little concern about this problem has been expressed.

The inadequacy of this program and the critical need for expansion of income and employment opportunities for older Americans received minimal attention during the 1978 Older Americans Act reauthorization hearings. Instead, attention was focused on a conflict between national contractors and state units over administrative control of the program and on eligibility requirements. Subsequently the two changes that were made by the 1978 amendments were those concerned with: (1) instituting procedures to assure that programs operated by the national contractors are coordinated with those operated by state units, and (2) assuring that Supplementary Security Income payments are not counted against eligibility in the program. Because the Administration on Aging houses, but has no administrative authority over, this program, it has not established specific goals to substantially increase employment opportunities for older persons, but rather has chosen to act as an advocate of the program in its present form.

Resources and Needs

What can be concluded from the pattern of resource allocation under the area planning and social services program?

First, resources for services are minuscule in face of need. The fiscal year 1977 appropriation for area planning and social services was $122 million, an amount considered grossly inadequate by many who testified on behalf of the Administration on Aging, and 1978 appropriations were $153 million. In view of the magnitude of the problems facing older people, particularly because of their poverty, it is difficult to believe that the total area agency expenditures (averaging less than seven dollars per older person per year) could have an impact. Even though their supportive services could be critically important in the lives of the small percentage receiving them, many elderly persons remain unaware and untouched by area agency activities—for example, only between twenty-five and thirty cents per older American was available in fiscal year 1977 to cover legal service and home repairs, and about fifty cents per person for transportation. As examples of this minimum effort, Congress found that "(1) approximately 3 per centum of the eligible population is presently served under community services programs authorized under [the Older Americans] Act, 17 per centum of whom are minority group members; (2) approximately 1 per centum of the eligible population is presently served by the nutrition program authorized under this act, 21 per centum of whom are minority group members" (*Congressional Record*, 1978, p. S11532).

Second, there is notable lack of congruence between the socioeconomic and demographic data, on the one hand, and gap-filling and supportive services, on the other. During the first two years of Title III implementation, empirical studies (O'Brien and Wetle, 1975; Steinberg, 1975; 1976) reported achievements with respect to building awareness of the needs of the elderly, mobilizing non-Administration on Aging resources, and increasing the number of elderly persons receiving service. Each of these studies, however, reported little congruence between the programs launched and the needs that had been identified by socioeconomic data and area surveys. In a recent national survey, transportation and income assistance were the two needs most often ranked by area agencies as having top priority within the planning and service area, yet the area agencies provided virtually nothing in the area of income assistance (beyond information) and little in absolute monetary terms in transportation (U.S. House, 1978e). The gap between the locally identified priority needs and the services funded under Title III were attributed by the area agencies primarily to insufficient funds (U.S. House, 1978e). And the Westat study found that in fiscal year 1976 transportation ranked first in number of area agency projects funded, with information and referral second, outreach third, and leisure and recreation fourth (Westat, 1978a, p. IV:18). A somewhat similar services profile for providers sampled in thirty-nine planning and service areas reported the types of services offered in 1976 in the following order: (1) information and referral (83 percent), (2) counseling (68 percent), (3) outreach (52 percent), and leisure and recreation (49 percent). Less than one third of the providers reported services in the areas of nutrition, housing, income, employment, home health, daycare, and legal and paralegal assistance (Westat, 1978a, p. III:18; Table 3–8).

The Westat research methodology and findings on area agency performance are significant in that they relate more to the improvement within the social service system of area agencies than to the primary needs of older persons. Westat reports increases in information and referral services and counseling services but does not correlate them with sociodemographic data or with needs as reported on by the elderly in the community. Although these linking and access services are consistent with the priority service areas mandated in 1975, they do not directly address the most urgent problems of the elderly. Many elderly who receive information and referral, for example, are not likely to be better off in terms of housing, income, or health as a consequence of receiving an agency referral.

Third, under the area planning and social services program, the political issues of equitable distribution and allocation of scarce resources are effectively rechanneled into attempts to reform bureaucratic fragmentation. Area agency patterns of service provision are predicated on the dubious assumption that the problems of the aged can be remedied by coordination, an assumption that found expression in the *Congressional Record*: "There is program fragmentation at the national, state, and local levels which inhibits effective use of existing resources, and coordination and consolidation of services allowing greater local determination to assess the need for services will facilitate achieving the goals of [the Older Americans] Act" (*Congressional Record*, 1978, p. S11532). Although Marmor and Kutza found "little evidence to support a direct-line connection between the stated problem—poor service delivery to the elderly—and the stated solution—better coordination" (1975, p. 13), the emphasis on planning and coordination continues to receive wide support (Westat, 1978a; 1978b; U.S. House, 1977e; U.S. House, 1977a). An earlier study of three hundred area agency directors found that only 26 percent believed that their first priority should be satisfying health and income needs. Instead, the first priority most agency directors recorded was setting up coordinated and effective services (Tobin, Davidson, and Sack, 1976, p. 22).

In recent years during the debate over income versus services strategies, a common assumption has been that retirement incomes of most older Americans are sufficient, that there is already an adequate income maintenance strategy (through Social Security), and that an intervention strategy concentrating on the more efficient use of resources through access services such as transportation, outreach, and information and referral will benefit all older Americans.

Since enactment in 1965, the Older Americans Act has been lauded by politicians, bureaucrats, and providers as a vital element in attaining the goal of a decent life for the elderly. Yet, what can Older Americans Act programs really do about the basic problems of income, employment, housing, health, and health care? Not enough, it would appear from the testimony of others who have examined the situation: "The statement of objectives set forth in the Older Americans Act is far broader than the authority given to the Administration on Aging in meeting these objectives. . . . for example, the inclusion of a requirement for suitable housing . . . is obviously an objective which the act has very limited power to accomplish directly since the major responsibility in the area rests with the Department of Housing and Urban Development. . . . the stated objective of an adequate income in retirement . . . is an objective which is far beyond the limited scope of the [Administration on Aging] to achieve" (Martin in U.S. House, 1977e, p. 71).

What, then, is the capacity of the Older Americans Act to resolve the large-scale problems confronting the elderly in the coming decades? While many within the aging network are content with expanding their own domain and interests, some policy makers have sought to examine the basic concept of the Older Americans Act from a long-range perspective. As Robert Benedict observed prior to his appointment as U.S. commissioner on aging, the area agencies do not have the authority or the capacity to foster change in the magnitude required to serve one American in ten today and one American in eight by the year 2000: "The system of area agencies, as marginal coordinating agencies and simple funding conduits probably will not be very successful. . . . these agencies are not in a position, they do not have the authority . . . the capacity or the resources to manage the change in the magnitude required to resolve the large-scale problems" (U.S. House, 1977e, p. 5).

Implementation Politics: No Villains, Just Victims

Having analyzed the shortcomings of interest group liberalism and the pluralistic ideology that provides support for policies determined by pluralistic politics, and having examined the eighty federal programs potentially benefiting the elderly, I want to explore why so few of the efforts seem to really benefit the elderly. Although I will examine why state and area agencies created by the Older Americans Act are unable to achieve the objectives for which they were created, I believe the problems identified may be applicable to many more policies and programs.

The politics governing implementation of the Older Americans Act have six primary sources or determinants. First, coordination engenders interorganizational domain conflicts and heightens interest-group politics, thus intensifying the survival, maintenance, and expansionary activities of the organizations involved. Interest-group politics and the resource consumption caused by the competition of organizations against each other prevent the concentrated deployment of available organizational resources toward the act's central objectives. These tendencies increase significantly when resources are scarce.

The second determinant of implementation politics is the inadequate resource base available under current decentralized social policies. Federal, state, and local funding for urban services is shrinking at precisely the same time as the service demand is increasing. The larger context of Older Americans Act politics is one characterized by the increasing scarcity of, and competition for, resources for social services and by the improbability of developing comprehensive, coordinated service systems under market conditions dominated by private enterprise. This situation is aggravated by the proliferation of federal, state, and local programs and their administrative and fiscal fragmentation.

Third, the public access to and greater involvement in human services issues renders the politics of human services far more vulnerable to goal-displacing conflict than the politics that impinge on the economic sector. This structural conflict occurs because the agencies established by the Older Americans Act operate in the public sector. As argued by Friedland, Alford, and Piven (1977), the most vulnerable public sector social services are likely to be those that deal with problems of the disadvantaged (for example, the aged). Human services are open to more public scrutiny than are government activities relevant to the economic sector—regulatory bodies and such indirect mechanisms as tax policies shield activities of this sector from view. For example, employers and employees receive a multibillion dollar federal tax subsidy when private health insurance is purchased by employers as a fringe benefit for employees.

The result of this split between the human services and economic sectors is the structural segregation and insulation of agencies that in effect create social problems from the agencies responsible for treating those problems. Health insurance again provides a good example. The Treasury Department, through the tax policies established in Congress, fosters the purchase of private health insurance, which leads to an excessive use of medical services that in turn drives up the costs of health care and fuels inflation. But the Department of Health, Education, and Welfare, in trying to put a cap on rapidly rising medical care costs, is helpless to do anything about tax policies that subsidize one of the major forces contributing to the problem. Discontent about ineffective policies is likely to be directed against the agencies that manage the problem rather than those that might have some leverage in altering the conditions that created it (Friedland, Alford, and Piven, 1977, p. 16). In and of itself, this segmentation of the problem from the solution prevents alleviation of the problem.

Public agencies dealing in social services and human misery are both the most politicized and the most likely to be neutralized if serious efforts for change are mounted. The most depoliticized are those activities that relate to economic development and the regulation of the public and private economy, for they are structurally hidden from public view. Thus, the Department of Health, Education, and Welfare is attacked by the medical, hospital, and insurance lobbies for its effort to control costs, but little is said and nothing is done about the federal subsidy for private health insurance.

The fourth source of implementation politics under the Older Americans Act is the very complexity of the problems of the aged. These are so numerous and interrelated that there is little clarity about how to design and carry out implementation strategies that will work. In such cases of uncertainty, two tactics are likely to characterize program planning and development (Estes and Freeman, 1976). One tactic (and one form of intentional ambiguity) is to avoid stating with specificity the guiding perspective that is linked to a particular effort. An example of such an approach is recreational programs, which are widely assumed to be beneficial but do not seek specific outcomes for the elderly; to do so would require commitment to a theory concerning the cause and effect of their problems. Another tactic to deal with a complex problem is to create broad-scale comprehensive innovations and interventions in which there are a large number of inputs with many vague objectives. The 1973 area planning strategy under the

Older Americans Act exemplifies this second tactic. The approach is similar to that of a physician who treats a patient with multiple complaints by means of multiple drug therapies simultaneously. Even if the patient improves, the doctor cannot duplicate the results in other patients. Opposition to comprehensiveness in human services may sound like heresy, but if we are to know what the actual impact of intervention efforts and federal policies is, it is necessary to know what efforts produced what consequences. At any rate, both tactics have resulted in program uncertainty and the conflict and politicization attendant on such organizational uncertainty.

The fifth source of implementation politics is decentralization, the backbone of the area planning and social services programs as represented by a system of state and substate planning agencies. The Administration on Aging, which administers these programs, oversees state units on aging in their development of area agencies, nutrition projects, and a number of other Older Americans Act programs. This aging network includes multiple jurisdictional areas, some of which are geographical and some political. Overlapping a diverse range of administrative and political activities, the network lacks both programmatic and jurisdictional coherence at state or local levels (Estes and Noble, 1978). Until the 1978 reauthorization bill, projects in the same locality that were funded under different titles of the Older Americans Act were not even necessarily coordinated with designated priorities under the area plan set by the area agency.

The sixth source of implementation politics results from the ambiguous goals sought through the network of agencies created by the Older Americans Act. The implementation of the act necessitated the creation of bureaucratic structures at the federal, state, and local levels. Bureaucratic organization is an effective form of control when the program tasks are routine and clearly specified and the inputs and outputs can be easily measured (Weber [1922], 1946). Bureaucratic dysfunctions arise when the given tasks or goals are ambiguous, thereby permitting staff to use discretion in the timing and method of accomplishing specified tasks and routines. Because planning, coordination, and pooling are vague strategies, the bureaucracies implementing them may alter the intent of programs through their interpretations. The administrative promulgation of rules and guidelines by the Administration on Aging is the major way in which the area planning and social services programs are clarified. This control over the regulatory process provides the Administration on Aging and its allied state units with significant power in directing the implementation process. It also renders them subject to intense but counterproductive conflicts over interpretations of policies. Under such conditions of ambiguity, uncertainty, and conflict, major goal displacement regularly occurs at all governmental levels, with the Administration on Aging, state units, and area agencies embroiled in conflicts over the direction and content of their programs (Estes, 1972; 1974a; 1975a; 1976a; Estes and Noble, 1978). But all of this bureaucratic maneuvering seems to take place at a great distance from the elderly themselves, who still face the same problem of inadequate income and all of its consequences that they faced long before the aging network came into being. As Binstock (1978, p. 1814) observes, "Most of our public policies are not designed as interventions to solve social problems. Rather, they are enacted and implemented by public officials in a fashion likely to solve the problems of public officials."

Carroll L. Estes
Maureen Noble

VII

Accountability, Bureaucracy, and the Older Americans Act

━━━━━**:O▭O**━━━━**:O▭O**━━━━

> *Unable to evaluate whether the broad societal goal has been attained, program administrators [of the Older Americans Act] are turning to an evaluation of the strategy instead. They ask whether attempts at coordination have indeed resulted in a more 'coordinated' system . . . and so on. . . . The decision to evaluate only the strategy points to an important dilemma for government in general: if our strategies continue to be thus unrelated to our objectives we will be unable to be accountable to the taxpayer when we do not meet those objectives* [Brinnon, 1975, p. 4].

Older Americans Act agencies share with other human services institutions the problem of accountability. Social services, medical care, and education are criticized because they are consuming increasing amounts of the public's money with results that seem harder and harder to measure. Because of the difficulties in measuring even such outcomes as improved health status from a medical service or improved reading ability following an educational program, institutions are turning to measures of process to assess performance. Pupil/teacher ratios and class size are easy to mea-

Note: This chapter is based on Estes and Noble, 1978.

145

sure and record. So are the number of visits to a hospital emergency room or the number of nurses required in an intensive care unit. Moreover, if the effect of particular services on individuals is difficult to determine, even more difficult to evaluate is the impact of a program on a group or the population as a whole. What has been the effect of the Medicare program on the health status of the aged? Of the Elementary and Secondary Education Act on student performance?

When evaluation of effect and impact are so difficult, how is it possible to hold agencies and institutions accountable? Or, more specifically, how is it possible to determine who is accountable for what in human services programs supported with public funds? To probe these questions as they relate to the Older Americans Act, we found it necessary to examine not only the nature, scope, and sources of information used by the Administration on Aging but also the ways in which such information is used by agencies from the federal to the local level.

The term *accountability,* as used here, means the capacity to explain what actions have been undertaken and what resulted from those actions. It goes beyond fiscal monitoring or input-output reports; it requires an analysis of the effect, the effectiveness, and the broader impact of a program as well. Accountability requires that reliable and valid knowledge be made available for administrative and policy decisions concerning program expenditures, activities, and consequences and that the processes by which various outcomes are obtained be spelled out. In terms of the aging enterprise, accountability involves the public, the elderly, and their political constituencies, as well as the Administration on Aging, state and area agencies on aging, umbrella agencies, nutrition project agencies, and designated contractors and subcontractors with diverse perspectives, interests, and roles.

The Older Americans Act creates multiple problems of accountability, which can be traced to its intentional ambiguity, to interest-group politics, and to decentralization of policy and program decisions. Not only does the act have multiple and conflicting objectives, contradictory causal theories underlying its policies, and wide latitude for administrative interpretation, but it also requires agencies to be accountable to multiple governmental jurisdictions at the local and state levels. For example, an area agency on aging may be accountable to several municipal and county governments and to several private agencies, as well as to a state unit on aging. It is rare when an area agency is accountable only to a single city-county government. Similarly, state units are answerable to one or more agencies of state government, the Administration on Aging—including its regional offices—and Congress.

Materials released from the Administration on Aging, the federal Council on Aging, and Congress often use the term *aging network* to denote the arrangement of state units, area agencies, nutrition programs, senior centers, and other Older Americans Act agencies throughout the nation. The term implies that there exists a set of clearly differentiated roles and responsibilities resulting from the rational devolution of authority from national to local levels. In actuality, the network, with its multiple constituent agencies representing various geographical and political perspectives, is fraught with jurisdictional disputes and conflicting interpretations of respective responsibilities. The more than three thousand heterogeneous agencies funded under the pre-1978 Title III and Title VII are administratively decentralized and lacking in programmatic unity at the national, state, and substate levels. The growing acceptance of the network concept obscures the very cleavages that create many difficulties in accountability. The multiplicity of individuals and organizations involved, the complexity of disseminating and retrieving information through the network, and the time involved in clarifying ambiguous policy statements and instructions—each of these contributes to inconsistent policy interpretation at all levels. Thus, independent, but not always interdependent, units of the network are individually and jointly subject to stress from within and without. The problem is further compounded by the demand placed on this multitude of agencies to handle complex information flows and by the reporting requirements of the Older Americans Act.

Accountability may be based on contractual and legally binding arrangements or it may stem from the presumed intent of Congress rather than the specific language of a law or regulations. More often, it represents some mixture of these two. The information required for accountability to the Administration on Aging cannot be provided by current reporting systems, which focus largely on what can be counted and reflect a limited perspective on whether the basic intent of the Older Americans Act is being carried out. This problem, of course, is present in all levels of government. What can be measured (for example, how many services are provided, how much money is spent) becomes the unit of evaluation, without regard to the outcome of the service provided, unless it is easily measured. Unfortunately, the current national system of program accounting and evaluation for the Administration on Aging has structural and methodological problems that prevent a fair assessment of the efforts and activities, let alone the effectiveness, of Older Americans Act agencies. To develop program accounting and evaluation methods for a nationwide system of comprehensive services that must answer to many masters may well be impossible.

A program effort aimed at attaining national goals, yet widely decentralized and diversified in its efforts, creates thorny dilemmas of accountability. Policy differences and uneasy compromises between Congress and the executive branch over the years contributed to a national strategy for aiding the elderly that is neither internally consistent nor specific. Additional constraints on the Administration on Aging are its staffing reductions and its administrative location within another agency with multiple purposes— the Office of Human Development Services in the Department of Health, Education, and Welfare. These factors impede efforts to achieve national, state, regional, and local accountability.

Administration on Aging Staffing. The Administration on Aging has been hamstrung in its ability to assist state and area agencies to develop better systems of accountability because of staff reductions and transfers of functions and staff to its umbrella agency— the Office of Human Development Services—within Health, Education and Welfare (HEW). The staff reductions in recent years have resulted from decisions by the Office of Management and Budget and by the secretary of HEW, while at the same time Congress was increasing the Administration on Aging's appropriations and the number of separate grant-in-aid programs it administers. Between fiscal years 1973 and 1975, appropriations grew slowly, from $200 million to $245 million. The staff of the Administration on Aging remained relatively stable, declining only from 122 to 120, and the programs administered remained essentially the same.

Between fiscal years 1975 and 1977, however, appropriations increased from $245 million to $401 million and programs grew in number from five to seven, while the staff was cut from 120 to 102. Although appropriations exceeded $500 million in fiscal year 1978 and commitments were made to restore staff cutbacks, the number of staff positions available has never been restored to the 1973 level.

Throughout its life the Administration on Aging has existed within larger welfare and social services agencies in HEW. In 1973 it was placed in the newly created Office of Human Development Services with the commissioner on aging retaining authority in many areas. Its placement in that office has limited the Administration on Aging's programmatic and administrative latitude; it does not, for example, control its fiscal and staffing allocations. One consequence of these limitations is the current staffing shortage in the Administration on Aging. While the Office of Human Development Services staff members and offices perform necessary Administration on Aging functions, utilizing positions allocated to the Administration on Aging, expanded responsibilities under the Older Americans Act require increased staff with direct administrative responsibilities. The extent of the current staff shortage has been estimated by the Gerontological Society to exceed 30 percent of minimum requirements. Congress should make explicit who has the responsibility for program management and then allocate adequate staff positions for the Administration on Aging or the Office of Human Development Services to do the job properly.

Dilemmas of Decentralization

Although predating special revenue sharing, the Older Americans Act reflected the new federalism principles in charging state and area agencies on aging with setting priorities in accord with state and local needs. This decentralization, however, has posed serious problems of accountability because of the discretion provided state units and area agencies in making program decisions. A major controversy has been whether transfers of authority under the new federalism strategy would result in more responsive and better planned programs at the state and local levels or would actually produce the opposite effect (Banfield, 1961; Estes, 1975a).

Unless specified mechanisms of accountability are instituted, many are concerned that national objectives and priorities and the gains of the recent past may be lost with the devolution of authority from federal to local levels. For example, a spokesperson for the National Senior Citizens Law Center testified concerning the Older Americans Act's special emphasis on needs of low-income and minority older persons, reporting serious obstacles to implementation due to the ambiguous and conflicting language of the legislation. The representative of the law center said that the Administration on Aging "has no meaningful method with which to monitor the provision of Title III services to determine if the intent of the act is being met" (U.S. Senate, 1978a, p. 9). He recommended: (1) that the 1978 reauthorization require more complete and accurate monitoring of programs and services and that special statutory service preferences be strengthened; (2) that new regulations be promulgated, which would be more consistent with the intent of the act, concerning minority and low-income aged; (3) that meaningful reporting and monitoring procedures be required of area agencies; and (4) that regulations already in effect regarding states' responsibilities to monitor and assess the plans of area agencies be strictly enforced. This kind of legislative and administrative specificity is rarely achieved in human services programs. The law center's concern lends validity to Schultz's (1971) argument that incentives are central to achieving program goals. First, however, it is essential that program goals be sufficiently specific for incentive systems to be derived from them.

The primary dilemma of decentralization is in striking a balance between the state and local discretion necessary to plan for and meet the needs of the population, on the one hand, and the accountability required for determining if performance is congruent with national objectives, on the other. Warren (1973a) argues that the balance, of necessity, becomes a trade-off wherein accountability is sacrificed in the face of decentralization. He states that the trade-off occurs in standards, accountability and national social policy priorities. He concludes that the new federalism objectives of reducing red tape and paperwork through decentralization and grant consolidation are likely to be incompatible with national standards and accountability. Questions have also been raised about state and local capacity for planning and program decision making and the extent to which the removal of federal requirements will culminate in politically motivated, rather than need-based, programs and allocations (Estes, 1976c).

The Older Americans Act contains competing objectives, some short-range, such as those of the nutrition programs, and others long-range, as in certain aspects of the planning and pooling strategies. It remains to be seen whether the 1978 consolidation of the titles for area planning, senior centers, and nutrition programs will alter this. Because its short-term effect was visible and directly experienced by older persons, the nutrition program was credited as a great success, regardless of its long-term nutritional effects on older persons or its relative costs and benefits compared to alternative strategies for improving nutritional status (Estes and Freeman, 1976). Furthermore, because it provided a needed human service and was popular with recipients and because the number of meals and people served could be counted, the nutrition program was assumed to be accountable.

In contrast, the ambiguity of the area planning and social services objectives—which lend themselves to varied interpretations—have made state units and area agencies vulnerable to charges that they were accomplishing nothing because many of their required activities were not visible or immediate in their effects. Because their objectives were long-range, vague, and difficult or impossible to realize—such as coordinating a service delivery system—accountability was difficult to achieve. Measures for expected accomplishment were difficult to design, particularly when so little was known about what subcontracted agencies actually did. The multiple and divergent goals selected and the differences in resource availability and commitment have caused state units and area agencies varying degrees of difficulty. These variabilities in turn created measurement problems for which no procedures have been designed. Precisely because of the multiple goals of planning, pooling, and coordination, along with the divergent conceptions of what they should be, there were increased pressures for these programs to be made answerable. This raised the question about how to make a program based on long-run objectives answerable in the short run. This problem will not be lessened by the consolidation of the programs authorized under the old Titles III, V, and VII into a new Title III, as mandated in the 1978 amendments.

The necessity to devise performance standards under conditions of intentional ambiguity and decentralization has led to sharply narrowing the focus of accountability—for example, by converting it from accounting for broad-aim coordination/pooling goals to accounting for small surrogate efforts such as the number of requests for information and the number of referrals made. In this narrowing of accountability what occurs is the reconstruction of the intervention effort itself through the specification of appropriate activities and outcomes—those that will be measured or counted by monitoring authorities.

Positive outcomes and acceptable performances that are easily measured and at least moderately attainable are likely to be sought by the reporting systems that are devised. For similar reasons, a program's effect on individual aged persons or of its broad impact on the aggregate social condition of the elderly are just as likely to be ignored. Because such effects are deemed irrelevant, no data are obtained concerning them and no incentives can be provided for improving them. The Administration on Aging's solution to this problem has been to request each state and locality to set its own independent standards against which agency performance will be measured. These individuals state assessments are to be aggregated to produce national performance report data. Given the anticipated variability and self-selection in such standards, it will be difficult for the Administration on Aging to draw conclusions about overall performance of state units on aging.

An Uneasy Compromise. Only during its early years did the Older Americans Act reflect the shared views of a Democratic administration and a Democratic Congress. During the period from 1969 to 1977 a Republican administration advocated policies designed to strengthen the White House and weaken Congress, while Congress initiated legislative action that was opposed by the executive branch. President Nixon advocated new federalism, which, by decentralizing decision making, would prevent Congress from setting program priorities. Congress preferred the approach of federally mandated and categorical programs to meet national needs. The differing congressional and executive views are exemplified in the different amendments to the Older Americans Act. The 1972 amendments established a categorical, direct-service meals program of congressional origin, while those in 1973 set up a broad-aim and nondirect-service coordinative strategy, reflecting the interests of the Nixon-Ford administration. In 1975 Congress imposed four priority services under the Title III block grant program, thus undercutting the White House's original intent to allow states and local communities to make program decisions.

A dual Congressional and executive approach was sustained in the 1978 amendments. Based on developing comprehensive coordinated service systems, area aging programs, with the exception of the 1975 priority services, seek system impacts that are long-term in their generation. Conversely, the congressionally initiated portions of the Older Americans Act aim at more direct, short-term outcomes through providing services with relatively immediate impact on the lives of older people. It had been hoped that consolidation of the separate planning and direct service authorities would improve results and reduce conflict and overlap among programs. The 1978 amendments, however, did not deal with the basic problem of fragmentation. The competing Older Americans Act emphases represented in these divergent perspectives create severe demands on all accountability systems.

Existing reporting systems tend to emphasize short-term, highly quantifiable data; long-run effects of programs are not being measured. Undoubtedly, this emphasis on short-run program tracking has occurred because political necessity calls for demonstration that the act directly benefits people. This results in deemphasis of the long-range attainments of planning, pooling, and coordination and will likely encourage area agencies to shift emphasis to whatever short-term outputs are being measured, regardless of their long-term consequences. Area agencies will not have to demonstrate accomplishment in essential areas, since little in the accountability system addresses activities and results within the mandated long-range objectives of the act. The Administration on Aging's reporting system needs to be far more comprehensive than its present short-term objectives. It should include data and analysis useful for policy making, for arriving at clear expectations about short- and long-term efforts by state units and area agencies, and for establishing criteria for what is and is not acceptable performance by state units, area agencies, and service providers. These goals for the reporting system cannot be met, however, unless Congress and the White House agree to a more limited and clearly defined set of objectives for each of the programs authorized under the Older Americans Act.

From the Bottom Up:
The Uses and Cost of Data

Data are needed at all levels of programming and policy making—local, regional, state, and federal. Local projects need data for program management, monitoring, and assessment. The area agencies need data to monitor and assess the effects of area plans, funding decisions, and coordination and pooling activities. Ideally the agencies should not only monitor projects but evaluate outcomes; few, however, have the capacity to do this. The state units require data to assure performance and contract compliance, fiscal accountability, and uniform implementation of regulations. The Administration on Aging needs data on impact and performance of national program strategies for itself, as well as for the Office of Human Development Services, the secretary of Health, Education and Welfare, the Office of Management and Budget, the president, and Congress. Congress needs the information to make national policy and to consider alternative strategy decisions. Each of these administrative, program, and policy levels has sets of roles and responsibilbies, and each function requires specialized data.

The term *data* implies information systems, and information systems that are set up to provide accountability mean paperwork. How, after all, can a program be evaluated unless there is a written record of its activities? How can instructions and policies be conveyed by administering agencies unless they are transmitted on paper? How can the public, not to mention advisory groups and subcontracting service providers, know what is going on and what official goals are unless they obtain the necessary information from authorized sources? The Administration on Aging seeks nation-wide compliance with the broad objectives of the Older Americans Act. In state capitals, state units on aging develop statewide plans, drawing from local recommendations and performing important administrative and monitoring functions. The fascination with data, the ability to produce and disseminate large amounts of information by means of copiers and computers, and the insistence on credible, reliable, and quantifiable data for decision making has filled many government agencies with information addicts. Program managers are interested in concrete information because it may be useful for public relations, politically expedient to have on hand, needed for program planning, and potentially useful for evaluating services. Since it is not always clear what specific information will be needed in the future, broad information development acts as an insurance policy.

In 1977, at the request of the U.S. Senate Special Committee on Aging, we undertook a study of the paperwork requirements generated by the Older Americans Act (Estes and Noble, 1978). As the study began, it became immediately apparent that the purpose of the paperwork was accountability. We found that reporting requirements for the old Titles III and VII alone had resulted in the accumulation of more than fifteen million items of data to meet the federal requirements for contract compliance.

Faced by reporting requirements not readily understandable or that seek data difficult or impossible to obtain, state units, area agencies and subcontracting agencies may resort to guessing or to making up data to comply with a given deadline. The data compiled nationally by the Administration on Aging are based on statistics that may vary widely from agency to agency, locality to locality, and state to state, thus resulting in elaborate but noncomparable sets of data whose reliability and validity are questionable. As these data are aggregated from localities to the state level and from state levels into national figures, the inherent inconsistencies and errors become magnified. This process creates serious problems because these data form the basic system of information for program managers and high-level public policy makers in deliberations on program implementation and legislative authorization and revision.

Reports from the agencies move upward, while major policy issuances and instructions flow downward to the local service provider. All the basic data on Older Americans Act programs are, then, developed at the local level, and local staff, often part-time and paraprofessional, bear a large amount of the reporting burden. Of data collected at the bottom of the pyramid of agencies, predictably some is lost as the information is sifted up to top decision makers and thus some distortion takes place. Reporting requirements at the bottom of the pyramid are not appreciably less than at the top, yet the small contractors must also keep services flowing. Further, they must maintain massive in-house paper systems for report data. At this level, the main concerns are for fiscal accountability, efficiency, project ratings and assessment, and program impact evaluations. There are also immediate needs for substantive information to guide ongoing implementation efforts. Such data are not readily forthcoming because of lack of clarity regarding the goals of planning, pooling, and coordination; confusion about how to measure performance; lack of baseline data on the needs of older Americans or on the status of local resource development and commitment; and the unavailability of local project data, which are aggregated and summarized and thus not retrievable for project-by-project comparisons.

Performance Measurement and Compliance Documents. As a multiple-goal strategy, the Older Americans Act requires that measures of short-term, intermediate, and long-term performance be used to examine area agency effect on program development, interorganizational and power realignments and rationalization of resource allocations for services. This places a heavy demand on the limited resources and evaluation capacity of state units and area agencies. Also, efforts by the Administration on Aging to specify performance measures often overreach state and local capacity. An example is the recent effort to identify and develop national and statewide baseline data on the number of people served and of dollars expended on aging services. Since the collection requirements of such measures exceed the available time, money, and staff expertise of agencies, the data will be of questionable accuracy.

The Administration on Aging's 1976 program instructions initiated a "bottoms up" process whereby area agencies were asked to set their own standards, which would then be aggregated at the state level and used by state units, along with their own data, to set standards for state-level activities. The national aggregation of this diverse information, coupled with federal activities, is meant to constitute the national performance standards. Such delegation of authority for establishing criteria to judge a project's activities is consistent with the new federalism strategies mandated by Congress (Estes, 1976c). Of note, however, is the potential negative consequence of deemphasis on national policy objectives for the aged. Crucial here is the problem that a reporting system predicated on self-created standards and self-evaluated performance poses for accountability. It is difficult to specify who is accountable to whom and for what. It will be equally difficult to determine if national goals are realized with such wide variability in state and area standard setting.

Performance measures, when provided, focus on performance of local subcontractors and do not tap state unit and area agency performance. The focus of accountability is almost purely on service outputs of subcontracts; yet, service subcontracting is only a small part of area agency responsibility. An additional gap in this reporting system is that it obtains no information on processes by which programs are implemented and reflects none of the dynamics or problems of implementation within state units and area agencies. What is needed is not simple tracking of inputs (dollars) and outputs (contracts, services), which are easily quantified, but information on how programs work. The current compliance reporting system does not capture these processes and lacks the very data needed to guide regional, state, and national regulation and policy development, thus denying program managers at all levels the information necessary to understand how a preferred program outcome was (or could be) achieved. This flaw in accountability limits the Administration on Aging's knowledge as to what works and denies it the ability to modify existing strategies or design new ones.

In the case of the Older Americans Act, a system of control has arisen that emphasizes narrow administrative achievements rather than broad programmatic ones. Lacking clear operational definitions of ends to be reached, the accounting systems of the act emphasize the number and types of contracts and services, not the effects of these efforts, and they thereby constrain local initiative for long-range efforts. Political necessity encourages the Administration on Aging to use criteria focusing on immediate outcomes that yield report data rewards. Hence, agency leadership sets aside program and policy efforts of long-range import in favor of projects shaped by short-term program implementation politics. Many mandated activities no longer appear in the reporting system, and it is possible that valuable approaches within the larger strategies of the Older American Act become discredited simply because there are no data to prove or disprove success.

Accountability and Baseline Data. The availability of baseline data is a prerequisite for evaluating performance. But in programs as diffuse, decentralized, and complex as those authorized by the Older Americans Act, it is an enormous task to develop this data. An examination of the Administration on Aging's efforts to develop national baseline data for state units, area agencies, nutrition projects, and subcontract operations revealed no attempt to tap reliable and valid baseline information that would permit relevant comparisons of one project with another in terms of success of the project or effectiveness of program management in organizing resources. Project ratings based on output/outcome classifications that would differentiate between projects with similar objectives and demographic environments are necessary for decisions as to funding new projects or refunding older ones, but such ratings currently do not exist. The manner in which data are aggregated and reaggregated from subcontractor to area agency, to state unit, and then to the national level prevent any comparing of the relative success of different projects. (No records of individual project activities within states are forwarded to Washington, D.C.) Further, these reports tend to measure volume of business rather than program effect on the population served, severely limiting their utility.

Federal Accountability and Evaluation. The complexity of Older Americans Act goals, combined with multiple implementation strategies, decentralization, ambiguity, and local discretion, make evaluation and accountability almost impossible. The crux of evaluation is to distinguish a program's effects from those of other forces working in the situation. The components of program evaluation are: (1) the effort expended (amount of activity/input), (2) the effects (results of the efforts), (3) the adequacy of the impact, (4) efficiency (the effect in relation to the cost), and (5) the process (how it was achieved) (Suchman, 1967). Under the best of circumstances, rigorous evaluations are difficult for social interventions based on multicausal models. This is particularly true when, as in the Older Americans Act, such causal factors as planning, pooling, and coordinating are considered interrelated and requisite to achieving goals.

Although the planning, coordination, and pooling strategy appears logical, its complexity, along with the apparent inability of program managers to uniformly define outputs, impedes a national system of monitoring or evaluation. The overextended program design of the old Title III, for example, with its multiplicity of competing objectives, is impossible to evaluate except in relation to effort expended (Estes and Freeman, 1976). This accountability problem is compounded with the consolidation of the old Titles III, V, and VII into a new Title III, mandated by the 1978 amendments to the act.

Current evaluation contracts and plans for the old Title III and VII programs do not address issues of national-level program impact. This lack of central accountability produces uncertainty among Older Americans Act agencies about what should be emphasized (low-income or all-income elderly), how to concentrate scarce resources, and what constitutes acceptable performance for the major intervention strategies within the old Title III. Further, without knowing what represents an acceptable performance, how can agencies be held answerable? And, without clearly delimited long- and short-term expectations, how can the success or failure of Title III or Title VII be substantiated and assessed in comparison to other national strategies aimed at the basic objectives embodied in Title I of the Older Americans Act? It is not enough to examine each program or service individually. A number of broader questions and hypotheses need to be examined, including the assumption that area agencies are the only feasible means for attaining Older Americans Act objectives. Other potential vehicles, such as direct provision of services to areas without area agencies, should be examined. Such an approach would study samples of localities with and without area agencies for relative resource base development before and after the 1973 amendments. An evaluation of the old Title VII nutrition program should ask whether other program strategies could achieve the same or better results for the same or less cost. The national evaluation study of Title VII, currently underway, focuses on social, rather than health, benefits. Whether another approach could better achieve what the old Title VII accomplished has not been considered.

Much of the research supported by the Administration on Aging has been devoted to improving planning and coordination activities rather than to making comparative evaluations of programs or to questioning intervention strategies. Evaluations are needed that would address the relative effectiveness of different approaches employed within a national strategy. Whether the Administration on Aging could introduce planned variations into structural or programmatic requirements in order to test the effectiveness of different strategies should be examined. The use of such variations might in fact make it possible to determine whether the Older Americans Act in general and the area agency programs in particular are even assessable. It should also be possible to evaluate outcomes in specific program elements through studies of program elements, for example, the relationship between a pooling strategy and a certain type of client impact (Estes and Freeman, 1976).

The Older Americans Act reflects an accountability system that largely by-passes the act's effect on the twenty-three million older persons for whose benefit it was designed. Our investigation brought to light no past, current, or proposed research on the Older Americans Act from the viewpoint of the elder American. The crucial questions regarding the goals and beneficiaries of the act are:

1. Is there any difference, experientially, between what the lives of older persons are like today and what they were like prior to implementation of the Older Americans Act in 1965 or prior to the 1973 amendments? Individually? In the aggregate?
2. If the condition of older persons has in fact improved, what relationship does such improvement have to individual strategy components (or the totality) of the Older Americans Act?

3. To what extent have the goals of the Older Americans Act been achieved? What relationship, if any, have special Older American Act programs had to the achievement of the goals?

To answer these questions, studies are needed of samples of older persons selected from localities with varied area agency intervention emphases on advocacy versus planning or on services versus coordination compared with study samples of older persons from matched communities without designated area agencies or nutrition projects. Examination of local level distributional patterns of services for the aged prior and subsequent to the 1973 amendments would be useful, but unfortunately no data are available for such an evaluation. For example, there are no data on the level of service provision or unmet need in even a sample of localities prior to implementation of the 1973 Comprehensive Services Amendments (although it may be available idiosyncratically in some localities). Without such baseline data, it is not possible to accurately determine the effect of Older Americans Act agencies.

Major Compliance Documents and Accountability

Compliance documents provide an excellent means to assess the effectiveness of systems of program accountability. To make use of these documents, we visited a select group of state units, area agencies, area agency service contractors, and a Title VII nutrition project. We found that two primary objections to major compliance documents, as voiced by agency staff members who were interviewed, are their emphasis on administrative procedures and processes—that is, on how the agency will be run, not on what the agency will do; and the attempts of the reporting and monitoring system to make everything operational. Much information is lost because an area agency, a state unit, or the Administration on Aging wants everything reduced to bits of information.

We tried to test the validity of these objections by coding information in categories of administration, planning, services development, and advocacy. Data from the state unit on aging plan (a key document issued annually) make clear that 50 percent of the information collected focuses primarily on administrative agency activities and operations. This figure rises to 61 percent of all information in the state unit quarterly report and drops to 31 percent in the monthly fiscal report. In the state-level documents only 11 percent of the information addresses the combined categories of planning and advocacy. Taken as a whole, the information collection does not represent a balanced recording of state unit activities aimed at major mandates of the act (Estes and Noble, 1978). This holds true in area agency and nutrition project compliance documents as well. The area agency plan for fiscal year 1977 reflects a somewhat more balanced approach to information about key activities. However, this balance is not repeated in the area agency assessment procedures. The information of most interest to the contractor (in this case, the state unit) falls heavily in the area of administration—and the documents within the monitoring system reflect this emphasis.

The area agency subcontracting system's documents indicate the same interests. In the initial application stages, major portions of information relate to planning and services development. But at various points within the reporting system these emphases vary or disappear. Thus, information collected at the level of subcontractors reflects their major activity—provision of services. Except in the budget, the reporting system of the nutrition program under the old Title VII emphasizes administration and agency project operations rather than program development. Here again, the categories of planning and advocacy become residual, and since this information acts as a basis for major policy decisions at the area agency, state unit, and Administration on Aging level, its bias toward administrative procedures and organizational operations would be a severe limitation. It is possible, then, to document a trend within the system that emphasizes administrative procedures and activities and deemphasizes direct services development.

In considering the second objection—that the monitoring system attempts to make everything operational—we examined various types of information. Much of the data reflected the extent to which information was simply reduced to numbers. Multiple judgments appeared implicit in these assessment procedures, yet agency staff reported that they consistently experienced acceptance of their own clearly ambiguous data as objective, concrete, and valid reports of activities. This acceptance of program "guesstimates" by contract monitors was unsettling, especially since staff members at many different kinds of agencies indicated a desire for feedback, technical assistance, and evidence of genuine interest in program issues by their monitors.

The Value of Assessment Tools. Examination of the assessment procedures developed by the Administration on Aging revealed an emphasis within the system on quantifiable and descriptive information. In only a few instances were discrete bits of information drawn together to substantiate specific conclusions. The state unit quarterly report requires quantified data on services and program impact, but the passing up of such data from level to level has left the major qualitative information concerning planning, needs analysis, priorities, and service impacts of the area agencies and state units buried at the bottom of the pyramid. What arrives at the top is deceptively concrete in appearance—numbers served, dollars pooled, staff hired, dollars spent, and so forth. These are the data that appear in the state unit quarterly reports and reappear in the national summary of program performance.

A key document, the state unit objective assessment procedure, completed on a quarterly basis, contains 1,388 data items. Of these, 528 (38 percent) are assessment relevant in that (1) the objectives as stated were addressed without prior analysis of the standards for achievement or quality, and (2) the information centered on completion of identified action steps, without focusing on whether they actually forwarded the overall objective. The completion of a set of identified action steps is not in itself consonant with completing the stated objective. For example, a series of action steps focusing on documentation of need for transportation among elders may not result in an actual increase of transit services. Thus, document items that did not elaborate on the overall impact of the activity, on resources or services, were coded as useful for assessment.

Evaluation information identified in the major compliance documents was defined as information regarding actual outputs or impacts, not planned outputs or impacts. A meager portion of the total information collected in these documents could be identified as potentially useful for project evaluation. Concern that no one in Washington could possibly know what they were doing or what impact programs had, given the existing data reporting system, was evident among agency staff. They vigorously argued that absolutely no efforts had been made by the Administration on Aging to assess the mountains of data passed on in reports, and thus the data were not employed in decision making about the programs.

Information potentially useful for evaluation is not easy to develop and, given the scope of the Older Americans Act and the numerous mandates under which local programs operate, it is difficult to achieve impact measures that are not only fair in the short run (by capturing immediate impacts) and useful in the long run (in reflecting the complexities of impacts) but that also allow for ongoing evaluative comparisons over a period of time. Standards and baseline data are needed for making project evaluations. These must relate to expected productivity, acceptable contract performance, and impact. Such standards are difficult to develop and apply, particularly for Older Americans Act programs wherein the ambiguity of what planning, coordination, and advocacy actually are inevitably thwarts standard setting and performance measurement and often results in goal deflection (Estes, 1973; 1974b). In many direct service programs the standards are virtually created by the contractee who provides the service.

Problems with the Accountability System. From a methodological perspective the current accountability system has three major problems. First, no baseline data have been collected against which to measure the impact of the overall Title III area agency/state unit strategy. Effectiveness and impact cannot be properly evaluated without comparing the varied approaches within the general Older Americans Act Title III strategy or assessing changes in that strategy.

Second, the data, sifted up through the system, becomes progressively more quantified and less informative, thus providing less accountability. Units of services from distinctly different projects are grouped under such headings as home care or numbers served. Such data aggregation prevents comparisons at either local or state levels between different program designs and funding strategies. There is no way to compare even such simple data as costs per unit of service from one project to another. Within the funding parameters of the act, discrete comparative studies can and should be developed.

Finally, the utility of existing data for evaluation is questionable. The recorded data were repeatedly described by agency staff as generally unfaithful to what is happening. With no means tests or determination of participants' incomes, data on the number of low-income participants cannot be collected in a valid manner. Given the difficulty of maintaining unduplicated counts, minority participation cannot be accurately recorded. Overemphasis on quantifiable short-term activities, in a "get the numbers" attitude, yields scant incentive for targeting services to reach, for example, those who are homebound and handicapped, for this kind of approach would not yield large numbers.

Three state plans—the affirmative action plan, the training and manpower development plan, and the introductory statement of objectives—were examined for data development and information on these problems. Categories of information (administrative, planning, social services, and advocacy) and types of information (fiscal, quantifiable, descriptive, and analytic) were cross referenced with the data potential for assessment and evaluation. In all cases, less than half the information was coded as evaluation relevant.

Accountability: From the Top Down

A large flow of information from the Administration on Aging to state and local agencies, described by at least one recipient as "not immediately relevant to program operations, often fragmented, and open to misinterpretation," must be stored by these agencies because retrievable information is critical when regulations are changed. They must also make responses to specific requests, interpret laws and rules and issue new regulations. The sheer volume of this information creates a burden on all agencies, and its cost includes an enhanced potential for misinterpretation and error.

Four sets of issuances that originate with the Administration on Aging are the Program Instructions (PIs), Technical Assistance Memoranda (TAMs), Information Memoranda (IMs), and Memoranda from the Office of State and Community Planning (OSCPs). Based on an examination of one year's issuances, we estimate that an average of forty-four PIs are generated per year. These forty-four PIs require an annual total of 318 pages at a distribution cost alone of $64,276 for copying and $26,808 for mailing and envelope costs (at 1976 postal rates). This excludes staff costs in preparing, receiving, copying, redistributing, storing, and reading the information at the local level, as well as the tremendous costs for multiple copies at the state unit, area agency, nutrition project and subcontractor levels. Staff time for clarifying such policy issuances accounts for additional costs. For every federal policy requiring clarification, an additional 2,361 copies must be prepared and distributed to Older Americans Act agencies. In addition to the PIs there are a variety of TAMs, IMs, and OSCPs issued every year.

A major activity mandated by the Older Americans Act is ongoing planning. Since the 1973 amendments, planning has been emphasized in technical assistance materials and in basic instructions to state units and area agencies. These issuances from the Administration on Aging have covered: (1) advocate planning, (2) involvement of consumers and providers of services, (3) developing priority listings, (4) planning for program development and maximum utilization of existing resources, (5) long-range planning versus short-term planning, and (6) the role of needs assessments in the planning process. Recommendations to area agencies for developing area plans cover planning, the setting of objectives, and monitoring processes (Kirschner and Associates, 1975), all of which require large amounts of time and paperwork. The first phase of the planning cycle is focused on analysis of needs, resource inventories, and alternative courses of action. Then, once objectives have been set, the major planning function shifts to monitoring achievements that should produce data for restating or altering program objectives.

As area agencies and state units can testify, however, planning is not the only factor determining program objectives. Local planning priorities, in fact, are often subverted by political, fiscal, administrative, or jurisdictional considerations. Thus, the area agency planning process is largely unrelated to major decision-making processes affecting local resource allocations and priority programs, particularly those not represented among older Title III allocations. The effort, time, and money used for the area plan, which most agency members call a basic compliance and administrative monitoring document, appear to be an overinvestment in planning given the limited influence and control that the area agencies exert, and it should be reduced to a minimum. One would wish it were otherwise, but our study indicated that a disproportionate share of scarce area agency resources was devoted to these planning activities with very little to show as a result.

The issuance system presents additional problems. In particular it appears to be too unwieldly for promulgation and clarification of policy. Time lags in distributing PIs and TAMs, along with delays in clarification and follow-up at the local level, add to the general confusion and raise the question of whether the issuances are laws, regulations, requirements, guidelines, or suggestions. Some issuances appeared, in fact, to have reinterpreted policy. The value of the IM was also questioned by our respondents. Technical assistance communications are designed to stimulate state agencies to undertake expanded initiatives in basic programmatic activities. According to the Administration on Aging (1975), in every instance the purpose of communicating with the network is either (1) to convey mandatory policies and procedures or interpret or clarify policy questions to the network (binding PIs), or (2) to provide information (nonbinding IMs) and assistance to the network (nonbinding TAMs). Yet the new standards for national priority services in the state unit assessment tool (1976) and the planning process outlined in the "Instructions for Development of an Area Plan" reveal that TAMs may occasionally be invoked as policy.

Agency staff expressed concern that policy was being developed outside normal regulatory (that is, legislative) channels by means of PIs from the Administration on Aging and that the vague status of TAMs beclouds accountability because they are less than policy but more than information. Agencies report difficulty in distinguishing between these suggested standards and minimum acceptable performance standards. Thus, contract monitoring standards, priorities, and sanctions remain confused. An analysis of documents revealed the Older Americans Act, especially the old

Title III, to be vague as to specifiable objectives. At the same time, however, administrative compliance issues were sufficiently specific to restrict program flexibility and perhaps to sidetrack goal-oriented activity.

The Older Americans Act and Human Services

Compounding the difficulty in achieving accountability under the Older Americans Act is the larger problem of accountability in the human services as a general class. This problem has been considered by Silver (1976) and Foltz (1978) for maternal and child health programs and by Gartner (1977) for human services in general. Gartner argues that human services are "considered . . . a self-evident good," that often their consumption is mandatory, and that in many cases there are few alternatives to extant service providers systems. In addition, he calls attention to the sparseness of available performance information on human services and to the contention that collecting performance data "is too complex a process and . . . people would not be able to understand the results" (1977, p. 6). Gartner's general criticisms certainly apply to the Older Americans Act. Our analysis of the act showed, for example, that inadequate measurements of the effects and impact of services and other interventions severely restrict the capacity of administering agencies to impose external controls or to provide incentives to encourage preferred performance outcomes. Thus, problems of accountability under the Older Americans Act are a specific instance of the larger problem Gartner has described for the general class of human services.

Our findings as to accountability and the Older Americans Act are also corroborated by Hudson's recent study of the Title XX Social Security Act program. Characterizing Title XX social services as largely "permissive" in the degree of discretion afforded implementing actors, Hudson indicates that one of the results of this permissiveness is "lack of clarity concerning exactly who is responsible for what and where accountability ultimately lies. . . . (1977, p. 49). [There is] . . . multiple formal responsibility . . . [but] little effective accountability" (p. 52). Hudson's conclusions about Title

XX programs match our conclusions about the Older Americans Act.

I have mentioned to a number of congressmen the lack of specificity in the objectives of the Older Americans Act, and I have received a clear impression that this *intentional ambiguity* provides the Congress with leeway to counter criticism from constituents and the general public and room to move in some different directions from time to time. Further, this intentional ambiguity is fostered by the hierarchy of HEW from the top of the pyramid down because it obscures and protects policy (which can be made internally) from review or challenge.

With its mountains of data, the present reporting system actually has very little use except for fiscal monitoring. There are no indications that any efforts are made to assess these data aggregations. To make this reporting system useful for guiding regional, state, and national regulations and policy, the data should respond to clearly defined program goals and standards of performance—imposed from higher in the pyramid than the contractee. Baseline data on needs of the elderly and status of resource management and development should be retrievable for project comparisons and evaluation in order to guide ongoing implementation and provide information for decisions on project funding or refunding. Projections on impacts of planning, pooling, and coordination should be clarified from the national level.

In conclusion, note that issues of accountability, by definition, are not merely technical in their nature; they are ultimately political. This statement applies to accountability issues in general and to those of particular concern throughout this chapter. Accounting systems may be employed to advance the political positions and ideologies of program adherents or opponents. As such, the design and measures deemed appropriate and representative of acceptable performance may be highly political, both in their uses and their consequences.

Accounting systems may also be used politically to provide symbolic justification for a program or policy's continued existence. At the same time, accounting devices may protect programs and policies from challenge. With all the systematic bias of the accounting systems for the Older Americans Act (measuring short-term efforts numerically, and not measuring the potentially less effective indirect services), these same accounting procedures tend to defend the policies to which they apply; little direct challenge is possible because there is little data with which to make positive or negative judgments. In the case of the Older Americans Act, the vague, ambiguous, indirect services such as pooling and co-ordination are particularly well protected from substantive and substantial review by these accounting mechanisms. Without the possibility of accounting oversight as a basis for determining nec-essary policy modifications or shifts, the formulation of policy di-rections is left largely to bartering among the most organized and vociferous of interest groups that have the most to gain or lose from aging policies.

Although Older Americans Act programs are helping some older persons to live more satisfying lives by expanding service re-sources and thereby enhancing their well-being, my concern is that Congress and the responsible HEW officials cannot obtain a clear appraisal of the Older Americans Act efforts using current ac-countability methods. Nor can state and substate program directors confidently believe that they are feeding useful information into a system that provides trustworthy analysis of their reports, efforts and accomplishments. These data cannot inform major policy con-sideration of costs and consequences of alternative comparative national strategies. Nor can the data tell the President and Con-gress about the relative success of the diverse state and local ap-proaches to the Older Americans Act.

VIII

Decentralization and the New Federalism: Is the Solution Part of the Problem?

On the national level, new federalism has turned out to be a new hoax for the nation's urban centers. Emphasis on decentralization of program priorities and administration only makes sense if it is accompanied by commensurate resource increases to those areas with the most pressing needs. New federalism thrusts down program responsibilities without supplying the requisite funding levels [Silverman, 1967, p. 348].

Although originally enacted in 1965, when categorical programs and strong federal direction were dominant elements in public policy, the Older Americans Act has come to fit far more completely into the new federalism and decentralization policies that emerged in the 1970s. The idea that those closer to the people are better able to solve society's problems has been embodied in new federalism legislation, which provides for increased state and local

Note: Portions of this chapter are adapted from C. L. Estes, 1975a, pp. 150–157; and C. L. Estes, 1976c, pp. 141–147.

171

determination of problems and their solutions. New federalism programs are thereby expected to transfer power from federal bureaucrats, and to some extent from national legislators as well, to elected and appointed leaders and their staffs in the states and localities. The central aspects of this strategy are examined in this chapter: first, revenue sharing as a specific example of new federalism in action; and second, decentralization as a core principle of the strategy.

Revenue Sharing: New Federalism in Action

The major arguments given for the initiation of new federalism proposals in the form of revenue sharing were: (1) state and local governments needed fiscal aid because of their inability to continue increasing property and sales taxes or to raise other revenues in proportion to their increased expenditures; (2) a redistribution of federal revenues through revenue sharing would result in an overall increase in funding available for state and local programs; (3) growing administrative and programmatic fragmentation at the national level had made government programs less and less responsive to the needs of the population; (4) states and localities could allocate resources more effectively than could the federal government if they were given the authority to do so; and (5) the increasing and disproportionate concentration of power in Washington not only was expensive but also made bureaucrats insensitive to program needs at local and state levels (Beyer, 1974), and this in turn had created a growing antagonism to the federal government (Berger and Neuhaus, 1977).

Revenue sharing was the Nixon administration's major hope for slowing down the growth of federal categorical grant-in-aid programs and for redistributing political power from national policy makers to local ones. It also provided a means to shift power from Congress to the White House (Muskie in U.S. Senate, 1973; Nathan, Manvel, and Calkins, 1975; Banfield, 1971). Although the arguments favoring revenue sharing were challenged, legislation enacting the first new federalism program of major importance, the State and Local Fiscal Assistance Act of 1972 (commonly known as general revenue sharing or GRS), was signed into law in October

1972. In 1976, GRS was extended for another three-year period, which ends in 1980.

In assessing the impact of this and other new federalism legislation, it is important to realize that revenue sharing may be conditioned or unconditioned. Conditioned revenue sharing restricts the use of revenue-sharing funds to fulfilling some specified federal intent, requiring, for example, that states and localities be concerned with particular programs or goals that Congress and/or the executive branch deem to be in the national interest. Examples of conditioned or special revenue sharing are the Comprehensive Employment Training Act (CETA) and Title XX (social services) under the Social Security Act.

In contrast, unconditioned or general revenue sharing permits the unrestricted and therefore highly discretionary use of funds and provides state and local authorities with the power to use federal tax funds in ways they themselves devise. Approximately $30 billion of GRS money was authorized for expenditure between January 1972 and December 1976, when the act was originally scheduled to expire. The renewed authorization allows an annual federal expenditure of $6.85 billion; appropriations in the six years since enactment have ranged from $5.3 to $6.85 billion annually. Formulas employed in computing the amounts of funds distributed are both complex and controversial. They include computations based on: (1) population, (2) urbanized population, (3) per capita income, (4) state income tax collections, and (5) tax effort (the five-factor House formula); and computations based on (1) population, (2) tax effort and (3) per capita income (the three-factor Senate formula). The higher of these two amounts is selected for each state (U.S. Congress, 1973). Within each state one third of the funds are allocated to state governments and two third of the funds is allocated to state governments and two thirds to local governments, according to each state's formula,

The GRS funds provided under the first 1972 enactment were restricted only to the extent that they be used for (1) "ordinary and necessary capital expenditures" and/or (2) "ordinary and necessary maintenance and operating expenses" in any of eight priority areas—public safety, environmental protection, public transportation, health, recreation, libraries, social services for the poor or aged, or financial administration. Yet, because there was no requirement that these GRS monies be used for specific maintenance or operating expenditures in any of these eight categories, the expenditure priorities were virtually meaningless. Theoretically all GRS monies could be spent for capital expenditures.

The discretion afforded states and localities in GRS allocations was further extended under the 1976 amendments, which removed all priority expenditure categories, as well as the planned-use reports for GRS monies. Thus, GRS spending has become increasingly unconditioned. In spite of this flexibility for state and local officials, however, there was very little spending on new programs or for expansion of ongoing services (Nathan, Manvel, and Calkins, 1975), as has been the case with funds for ongoing services. The fact that GRS money initially was not viewed as permanent reportedly affected allocation decisions. More recently, the relatively insufficient funding levels of GRS (it provides less than 30 percent of the annual state and local budgets) are expected to further limit spending for both new and ongoing programs, particularly in the face of growing fiscal crises that have been worsened by the threat of taxpayers' revolts. Although GRS was billed by its legislative supporters as new money, it was widely feared that the sums available would not only vary over time but would not constitute new money at all. Many state and local officials have increasingly felt that this money will replace other sources of federal revenue and that, even with GRS, an overall *decrease* in funding assistance to states and localities from the federal level may well result (or that this has already occurred).

Some states and localities have fared poorly, compared to others, in terms of the total dollars available from GRS and other funding sources, partly because the formulae for computing revenue-sharing allocations do not account for the relative commitments of states and localities to services. These discrepancies and attendant fears about the instability and overall benefits of GRS also derived in part from the Nixon administration's large budget cuts immediately following the enactment of the State and Local Fiscal Assistance Act of 1972 and from enacted and proposed special revenue sharing programs that are meant to reduce and/or rechannel the flow of federal funds to states and localities.

The second major type of new federalism is conditioned or

special revenue sharing. As partially enacted, it merges a variety of categorical programs into functionally related areas. Special revenue sharing monies are to be used for limited purposes and to replace existing grant-in-aid categorical programs with block grants. In the case of human services, special revenue sharing allows almost unlimited flexibility to states in the choice of social service interventions, confining the role of the federal government to specifying national objectives for specific social services (Mogulof, 1973). Theoretically, special revenue sharing is a way of providing for goal determination at the federal level, while the determination of means is assigned to the local level. But, in the broad enactment of some major pieces of special revenue sharing legislation—for example, Title XX of the Social Security Act—state and local officials have been given choices for both goals and implementation. Although there was consolidation of a number of categorical health programs in the Comprehensive Health Planning and Public Health Service Amendments of 1967, the concept of special revenue sharing had not emerged clearly at that time. The act creating CETA and the Housing and Community Development Act were the first major pieces of special revenue sharing legislation. The most significant human services programs were authorized by Title XX of the Social Security Act in January 1975.

Any effort to assess the impact of new federalism for aging services must examine what effects the elimination of categorical grants would have on specific subpopulations. While some revenue-sharing programs include special mention of older persons, there are no guidelines or mandates to assure allocations based on levels of need. Nor are there mechanisms for tracking the funding allocations to the aged or other population groups specially mentioned. The general problems of accountability in federal programs are thus exacerbated by new federalism strategies. Also important is the fact that different general and special revenue sharing programs have different decision-making authorities, located at a variety of jurisdictional levels. Three types of revenue sharing can be distinguished: (1) programs in which funds are allocated to both state and local levels, with decision making about distribution at both levels (general revenue sharing); (2) programs in which funds are allocated to the state level only, with decision making about distribution mainly at the state level; and (3) programs in which funds are allocated primarily to the local levels, with decision making at the county and city levels. (See Table 6.) What is evident is that for certain types of programs state level advocacy is likely to be most efficacious. For some, organization on the city or county level is better. For still others, coordinated state and local effort is most likely to enhance success in obtaining resources for the aged.

Central and continuing issues surrounding new federalism programs concern their political, distributional, and fiscal effects, as well as the extent to which new federalism signals a withdrawal from national priorities, commitments, and standards. The redistribution of power among federal, state, and local officials that results from new federalism is an issue of major political importance. Equally important is the degree to which new federalism increases politically motivated, rather than need-based, determination of programs and allocations for services and thus augments the influence of special interests—especially providers—as opposed to political parties or broader-based citizen groups. Given almost complete discretion in determining the use of GRS funds, state and local officials are required to make highly political decisions. The accessibility of local politicians to local interest groups heightens pressures on them, rendering them more vulnerable to compro-

Table 6. Major Revenue-Sharing Programs Affecting the Aged: Governmental Level for Allocation Decisions

	Governmental Level			
Revenue-Sharing Program	*STATE*	*LOCAL*		
		County	*City*	*Township*
General revenue sharing	X	X	X	X
Community development (Housing)		X	X[a]	
Comprehensive Employment and Training Act		X	X[b]	
Title XX (Social Services)	X			
Urban Mass Transportation Act	X			

[a] Restricted to cities over 50,000 population.
[b] Restricted to cities over 100,000 population.
Source: Zucker and Estes, 1976, p. 36.

mise or corruption. In addition, because new federalism funding lacks the relative uniformity and restrictive input provided by categorical federal programs, it results in less necessity for state and local politicians to make compromises in the direction of broad national objectives. (Some political observers argued, however, that there would be less politics, fewer compromises, and fewer trade-offs with GRS because it would offer local officials the opportunity to strengthen their political positions by means of their discretionary authority over the spending of federal funds. See Banfield, 1971.)

The distributional effects resulting from the criteria and formulae employed in the allocation of revenue-sharing dollars to different types of states and localities and between states and their localities have been a cause for concern. It has been argued that the current formulae for GRS and special revenue sharing programs benefit wealthy states that do not have large numbers of poor or elderly residents. Many states and localities have reported that they have actually lost large sums of previously available program dollars because of the formulae for disbursing GRS money (Nathan, Adams, and Associates, 1977; Bach, 1977). These fiscal effects, as well as the difficulty in tracing the effects of GRS expenditures, have raised questions about how the effects and responsiveness of revenue-sharing programs can be evaluated and how much accountability should be required. It is asserted that the electorate will defeat state and local officials who are not responsive to local needs and that Washington bureaucrats controlling national programs are not required to be responsive because there is no electoral process by which to recall them. It is a somewhat questionable assumption, of course, that politicians who are unresponsive will be recalled. This presumes electoral awareness of the responsiveness, or lack of it, of state and local officials in their allocations of revenue-sharing monies—an unlikely situation given the complicated maze of revenue-sharing issues.

The extent to which new federalism programs signal a withdrawal from national priorities, national commitments, and national standards is another major cause for concern. Does this policy trend signal the closing out of categorical programs at the federal level? And if so, what would be the impact of such closures, not only on states and localities but more importantly on those who receive services from categorical programs. Is it important to distinguish between those state and local needs that are in some sense national and those that are not? Are there overriding areas and directions that must not be left to local bargaining systems—or perhaps to chance?

Accountability Issues. Changes made by the 1976 amendments to general revenue sharing focused on the accountability provisions—civil rights enforcement, public participation, auditing, and accounting. The discretion given state and local officials was extended by the elimination of prior prohibitions against using revenue-sharing funds to match categorical grants and by the elimination of the earlier priority categories. Recipient governments, however, are still required to submit a final report to the Treasury Department stating the amounts and purposes for which funds have been appropriated, spent, or obligated and showing the relationship of those funds to the relevant functional items in the budget. Further, the report must identify the differences between the actual and proposed use of such funds. A recipient government is required to publish in at least one newspaper the proposed uses of revenue-sharing funds, along with a summary of its proposed budget.

When the 1976 amendments eliminated the priority expenditure categories, a new set of reporting categories defined by the Bureau of the Census was instituted. The category "social services for the poor and aged" was eliminated and replaced with the negative and inclusive category "welfare." Although many policy analysts contend that these priority expenditure categories are of little use in determining the actual fiscal allocations of revenue sharing, the elimination of the prior reporting category makes it virtually impossible to systematically track program area expenditures for services for the poor and aged. Defined as expenditures for public assistance programs (including administrative costs), vendor payments, and direct payments to indigents, the welfare category includes medical, hospital, and nursing home care provided to the needy; it also includes amounts paid from state and federal grants for welfare purposes. Further, this new reporting system does not distinguish between health services and social services, since many health services expenditures can be incorporated under the welfare category. Also, there are no age-based data. Major information gaps are thus inherent in the reporting systems for the largest new federalism programs.

Prior to the 1976 amendments to the State and Local Fiscal Assistance Act, GRS reporting categories were basically the priority expenditure ones: however, the procedures for compiling data using these categories were not defined, and it was left to individual jurisdictions to determine how the data for the annual reports were to be calculated and reported. The resulting lack of comparability among reports creates serious validity problems similar to those of the Older Americans Act. The existence of two types of reporting forms also makes comparisons difficult. Large jurisdictions must report nineteen expenditure categories, while small jurisdictions (with populations less than twenty-five thousand) report only six expenditure categories. Another 1976 change in reporting requirements permits actual-use reports to be based on the recipient government's fiscal year, not the federal fiscal year. This significantly reduces the potential comparability of expenditure data for GRS funds across states and localities.

Another critical issue hinges on the interchangeability of federal funds with other monies, which makes it difficult to track the use of revenue-sharing dollars. Once dumped into large pools of general budget monies, GRS dollars can then be channeled into accounts from which local dollars have been withdrawn, thus obscuring the ultimate uses of federal dollars. Juster (1976) has confirmed the inaccuracy of actual-use reports as approximate measures for the expenditure of revenue-sharing funds, particularly for governmental units of over one hundred thousand in population. One solution he proposed was "to require more detailed accounting reports, covering all funds available to recipient jurisdictions in a fashion that would prevent the confusion caused by fund transfers" (p. 10). But even the imposition of accounting reforms would not make it possible to track the use of these funds for particular population groups. Concern over this issue prompted the Senate Special Committee on Aging to report in 1976 that it is "virtually impossible to accurately determine how much general revenue sharing money is being used specifically for aging-related purposes" (U.S. Senate, 1976a, p. 174). This difficulty has been attributed primarily to interchangeability as well as to the pre-1976 practice of combining social services for the poor and aged into one category.

Juster was unsuccessful in his attempt to determine the impact of GRS on population groups. He noted: "Almost all respondents were reluctant to pinpoint GRS program impact on particular population groups. . . . In consequence, there are virtually no data with which one can examine the apparent impact of GRS on different population groups, insofar as impact is measured by the incidence of programs across different population groups" (1976, p. 65). Thus, the question of who actually benefits cannot be adequately addressed. While many GRS critics charge that the program has operated to the relative disadvantage of the poor and elderly, evidence on this point cannot be ascertained. Indeed, not to require accountability was part of the basic ideology upon which the program was predicated; no strings were to be attached to the federal funds.

Accountability problems for special revenue sharing programs are at least as great as for general revenue sharing. There is no central federal office or agency to assemble, coordinate, or examine information about the impact of various special revenue sharing programs on specific target populations or about the total distribution of program funds. Accountability issues under Title XX social services are no less thorny, and at least two different views about the problem of determining the allocation of Title XX funds for services to the aged have been expressed. One study could find little data about the makeup of program recipients: "When Title XX was established, a set of Social Services Reporting Requirements (SSRR) was also initiated. These data are beginning to provide a picture of the pattern of service delivery across the nation. . . . SSRR, however, does have certain limitations. Most notably, services are not reported by age of recipients, but by the recipient's eligibility category. This means there is no national mechanism to determine how many elderly are actually receiving social services. [Further] . . . few states monitored the implementation of the [Title XX] plan. While budget review and supervisory control are the major management mechanisms used to monitor expenditure patterns, the process is rarely constructed to provide information in terms of the service provision pattern, or performance is not analyzed in this manner" (Benton, Feild, and Millar, 1977, p. 15).

The National Council on Aging expressed its concern in less uncertain terms: "We must first underscore the most blatant and inexcusable fault in the current Title XX program; namely the lack of age-specific data on program recipients which would allow us to evaluate the program more closely. In this instance, state flexibility only serves to obscure vital information. . . . We are reluctant to create paperwork burdens for Title XX administrators, but there seems to be no way of judging whether or not a state is meeting the needs of its eligible elderly in proportion to their number in total population. HEW must collect and report more specific data such as age, race, and sex on Title XX recipients" (National Council on the Aging in U.S. House, 1977f, p. 2). Partly as a consequence of these concerns about Title XX and partly as a result of our report for the U.S. Senate Special Committee on Aging on accountability problems under the Older Americans Act (Estes and Noble, 1978), the 1978 Senate reauthorization bill for the act requires Health, Education, and Welfare to review the Title XX program in terms of its relationship to the aged.

Allotment of Funds. Available data regarding GRS expenditures indicate that most of the early GRS funds were spent either for construction and other nonrecurring capital expenses or to provide tax relief. With the exceptions of public safety and education, social services received relatively minor support, and indications are that spending for such services may have dipped to even lower levels as increasing fiscal concerns have been felt by states and localities. For example, in 1973, the Treasury Department reported that only 8 percent of GRS spending (actual and planned) was on social services, even though states and local governments were pouring money into building projects and public safety programs. Only 4 percent of the $9.5 billion expended by the end of fiscal year 1974 had been allocated to services for the poor or elderly (U.S. Department of the Treasury, 1975). In early 1973, the Deputy Comptroller General answered an inquiry from Representative Claude Pepper concerning general revenue sharing allocations for the aged. This answer contained results from a sample of governments, "selected primarily on the basis of dollar significance and geographical dispersion," that had authorized GRS expenditures prior to July 1, 1973. The information indicated that "of . . . 218 governments, 28 authorized the expenditure of part of their revenue-sharing funds in programs or activities specifically and exclusively for the benefit of the elderly. . . . About two-tenths of one percent of the total funds [were] authorized for expenditure by the 218 governments [for services for the aging]" (U.S. General Accounting Office, 1973).

Although some of the reports mentioned above are now five years old, they seem to have forecast the future. Only 2 percent of the GRS expenditures for fiscal year 1975 were reportedly allocated to social services for the poor and aged. Of more than $7 billion in GRS funds allotted between July 1, 1974, and February 28, 1975, only $6.1 million (less than 1 percent) were directed toward programs for the aged (U.S. Senate, 1976a). This led the Senate Special Committee on Aging to comment: "Our older Americans are still clearly not getting their fair share. Americans over sixty-five represent 10 percent of the population and 28 percent of Americans living below the poverty level" (U.S. Senate, 1976a, p. 175). The fifth annual report of the Office of Revenue Sharing (U.S. Department of the Treasury, 1978) reported a 3 percent expenditure for social services for the aged and poor during the period of July 1, 1976, through December 31, 1976. The largest single categories of expenditure were public safety (26 percent) and education (22 percent). During a roughly comparable time period it was estimated that $13 million of general revenue sharing funds were pooled by state units on aging in forty-seven states during fiscal year 1977 (Administration on Aging, 1977). Calculated on a base of $6 billion, the proportion of funds for older people remained less than 1 percent. The community development block grants tell the same story (see Chapter Five). For fiscal year 1976 only $18 million of an estimated expenditure of $2.34 billion could be identified as going exclusively for activities for the elderly (U.S. Senate, 1977).

The extent to which state units and area agencies have

sought and obtained revenue-sharing dollars has been the subject of several studies funded by the Administration on Aging. The pooling or drawing in of state and local resources has been a major mandate of the area agencies on aging created under the 1973 Comprehensive Services Amendments. Although state units have had the central role of advocate for the aged at the state level, they have experienced heavy administrative demands as a result of their mandate to designate and oversee area agencies in their states. The concentrated effort required for these tasks raises the question of whether state units have the resources to pursue revenue-sharing allocations, and similar questions arise for area agencies.

The Administration on Aging's major evaluation of area agencies indicates that general revenue sharing was available to only 14 percent of the probability sample of thirty-nine agencies studied (Westat, 1978a; 1978b). Steinberg (1976) also found that area agencies generated limited amounts of revenue-sharing income, although 28 percent of the agencies that he studied reported some general revenue sharing funds. More significant is the relatively limited dollar amount of funding received. Westat (1978b) found that the median budget for area agencies from revenue sharing was $15,000, with a range of funding from $1,000 to $150,000. A slightly higher percent of area agencies (22 percent) reported funding from Title XX. The median amount of Title XX funding was $61,000 and the funding range was from $40,000 to $516,000 (Westat, 1978b). Thirty-nine percent of the area agencies reported CETA funds and 11 percent UMTA funds. The dollar amounts of these funds ranged from $5,000 to $85,000 (median $40,000) for UMTA.

Looking at the figures another way is less encouraging. Sixty-one percent of the area agencies reported no budget resources from CETA; 78 percent reported none from Title XX; 89 percent reported no UMTA monies; and 81 percent reported no other federal sources of funding. Gilbert and Specht's study (1977) on Title XX found that 33 percent of the area agencies surveyed received some of their funds from Title XX, and that an estimated 50 percent did not even attempt to obtain their portion of Title XX funds. For those area agencies actually requesting Title

XX funds, 84 percent were successful. The most highly accepted
and successful of area agency efforts was the enlistment of public
officials, particularly at state and federal levels.

Additional studies of state unit and area agency involvement
in Title XX social services decision making indicate increasing activity of these agencies from a low pre–Title XX participation-
influence rating of 1.9 for state units and 1.5 for area agencies, to
post–Title XX ratings of 2.6 for state units and 2.4 for area agencies on a five-point scale (Benton, Feild, and Millar, 1977). Although showing improvement over time, state unit and area agency
scores do not compare favorably with similar ratings for state officials (2.8 to 3.0), other state agencies (3.0), service providers (3.2),
or even client groups (3.0)—all of which also show increases in
participation influence in pre– and post–Title XX comparisons.

Urban Institute studies on this topic report that, although
the elderly (sixty-two and older) make up 12 percent of the total
population, only 7.8 percent of Title XX services go to persons
eligible for Supplementary Security Income (SSI). The SSI-aged
comprise 7.6 percent of the total categorically related population,
while they receive   7.8 percent of the services for that population
(Benton, Feild, and Millar, 1977). (See Chapter Five.) The authors'
characterization of these data as evidence that some form of equity
has been achieved for the aged through Title XX appears unwar-
ranted and optimistic, particularly in view of the higher incidence
of poverty among the aged. The significance of the question of
equity for the aged cannot be overestimated. Although Title XX
is widely heralded as "the chief source of funding for social services
in the country and within each state" (U.S. Senate, 1977, p. 79), it
is also true that "the elderly do not fit squarely into the needs design as established by Title XX. The elderly often cannot be ab-
sorbed back into the work class, which is the major philosophy of
Title XX: to keep the individual off welfare and fit for gainful
employment. Therefore, the elderly clientele are forced to utilize
a wide array of services for indefinite periods of time with no relief
in sight. The justification and need for such services are obvious"
(p. 81).

The National Council on Aging has noted that the elderly

historically have not fared well in competition with other groups—children would be one example—for limited social services. This has been particularly true of those in greatest need, who are seldom able to ensure their own participation in service programs. The evidence is strong that this pattern persists. Even though Title XX was heralded as a new social service system, it has in fact been a continuation of the system existing prior to the enactment of Title XX. The council's view is supported by an analysis of the fiscal year 1977 Comprehensive Annual Service Program (Title XX), which revealed that "almost 60 percent of Title XX expenditures will be for services directed to children. Almost one fourth, 24.1 percent of expenditures, were to go to child daycare compared to only 1.3 percent to adult daycare. Under the universal services (provided without regard to income), 8.1 percent of total Title XX funds were spent on protective services for children; only 1.6 percent on such services for adults" (National Council on the Aging in U.S. House, 1977f, p. 3). Again, the first-year evaluation of the implementation of Title XX revealed that in most states the percent of Title XX services to SSI-aged recipients is below the percent of aged in the population. In some states, it is half or lower; however, 7.2 percent of all Title XX social services go to SSI-aged recipients (U.S. Senate, 1976a).

In his testimony before the Senate Special Committee on Aging, Secretary Califano found cause for optimism in the fact that in 1977 state and area agencies were successful in pooling more than $440 million dollars of cash and in-kind resources (Califano in U.S. House, 1978a). As reported by the Senate Special Committee on Aging, of the $440,403,806 pooled, $226,706,536 were cash resources. The dollars pooled came from Title XX (social services), Medicaid, CETA, general revenue sharing, Public Health Service programs, Economic Opportunity Act programs, Community Service Employment (Title IX of the Older Americans Act), and other programs (see Table 7).

It is worth observing that, even if the above figures are accurate—a questionable assumption—it would mean that between $19 and $20 per American aged sixty-five and over have been pooled from other federal programs, many of which are already

Table 7. Pooling of Funds by State and Area Agencies

Federal Program	Dollars Pooled
Title XX of Social Security Act	$77,135,326
Medicaid	33,314,309
Comprehensive Training and Employment Act	25,647,605
Housing and Urban Development programs (excluding community development)	22,780,041
General revenue sharing	13,401,457
Title XX nutrition programs	11,487,559
Public Health Service programs	11,366,978
Title IX of Older Americans Act	11,177,753
Community Development Act	11,113,706
ACTION programs	10,640,810
Department of Agriculture commodities	9,297,328
Food stamp program	5,156,645
Capital assistance grants (Department of Transportation)	4,966,150
Economic Opportunity Act (senior opportunity and services)	4,212,354
Legal Services Corporation	2,514,842
Economic Opportunity Act	2,297,592
Department of Transportation programs	1,696,571
Rehabilitation Service Act programs	1,626,711
Federal Energy Administration	1,518,729
Law enforcement assistance programs	690,615
Economic Opportunity Act (community food and nutrition)	648,912
Other federal programs	47,913,599

Source: U.S. Senate, 1978b, p. 121.

required by law to provide services to the aged. A more detailed examination of these pooling data raises further questions. The $33 million of Medicaid funds pooled represents less than 0.3 percent of the $16 billion in Medicaid expenditures; the $25 million of CETA pooling is a mere 0.2 percent of the $12.1 billion available nationally for fiscal year 1977; the $11 million of the Community Development Act funds is 0.5 percent of the $2.3 billion available nationally; the $13 million of GRS funds for the aged is less than 0.2 percent of the $6.8 billion available; and the $77 million of Title XX, along with the $11.5 million of Title XX for nutrition programs, is approximately 4 percent of the $2.5 billion of Title

XX funds—which is heralded as providing the major funding for social services in America.

The problem is not just a matter of priorities. Discrimination against the aged is widespread. The Civil Rights Commission's 1977 report on age discrimination revealed that the aged are victims of widespread inequities in all ten of the federal programs it studied. These inequities are embedded in federal, state, and local policies and procedures. Reporting that "we are shocked at the cavalier manner in which our society neglects older persons who often need federally supported benefits and services" (U.S. Commission on Civil Rights, 1977, p. ii), the commission went on to document systematic discrimination in the programs studied. Given such institutionalized barriers to receiving services, the problems that the aged face in obtaining their basic entitlements are more pervasive than is generally acknowledged. The pooling successes of Older Americans Act agencies pale in the face of the shocking unresponsiveness of American social institutions. This larger view of the problems of aged Americans makes clear that state and area agencies themselves are deluded by their belief that they can take more than minuscule steps toward attaining their assigned goals.

I remain both skeptical and concerned. Reliability and validity questions are particularly worrisome in relation to reports on dollars pooled. Despite Secretary Califano's optimism, moreover, my early concerns about the potential success and ultimate outcomes of new federalism programs for the aged and other disadvantaged groups have not been assuaged by the data. As I expressed it in 1976: "Current nationwide evidence provides no reason to think that the large majority of [state units] or [area agencies] would fare well if federal monies for social programs were entirely allocated at the state and local levels among competing interests (that is, without the fixed federal funding of categorical aging programs at those levels)" (Estes, 1976c, p. 146). As a consequence, "The more realistic and potentially dangerous result of backing off from national objectives with unconditioned revenue sharing [is that,] for whatever reasons, when released from federal requirements, programs for the elderly may indeed slip into oblivion . . . under such a new federalism strategy. This is . . . probable . . . because support for aging programs has to be renegotiated with advocacy efforts in each of the more than 39,000 individual jurisdictions which receive revenue sharing funds" (Estes, 1976c, p. 145).

Decentralization

Two crucial questions about decentralization are: Decentralization to whom and for what? Lowi (1971) argues that the decentralization of power to localities functions primarily to remove the policy process from the focus of large national movements, resulting in a transfer of public conflict to private arenas in which national movements have little influence. What occurs is the conversion of critical moral issues and goals into negotiable and administrative ones. Lowi argues persuasively that decentralization tends to plug government into the interest-group system. The result is maintenance of the status quo.

The popularity of the notion of decentralization may be traced to a basic American fear of the power of the state and a belief that each decentralization of government power is accompanied by an expansion of the mechanisms of representation. Theoretically, decentralization provides for expanding public representation, participatory democracy, and popular local control. In actuality, decentralization has tended to increase the influence of private interest groups because such influence may be more freely exercised when there is a reduction of national directives and oversight. Further, decentralization tends to foster the development of a particular type of interest group, the trade association, which attempts to establish regularized relations among possible competitors in the same industry, trade, profession, or economic sector. The more decentralized an activity, the more trade associations are necessary in order to protect those interests that might be compromised through decentralized, nonnational activities and perspectives. Such trade associations seek ultimately to replace open competition with closed administrative processes in which they work jointly with government in making key decisions. Lowi (1971) argues that trade associations are pernicious for democracy because they remove value questions from public view and settle them privately, with the support and collaboration of government officials.

The Older Americans Act and the decentralization principles embodied in it provide just such mechanisms for the devolution of responsibility for policy making from the governmental
to the private sector through interest-group pluralism. Old age
policies are now mediated in important and largely unknown ways
by such trade associations as the National Association of Area
Agencies on Aging (NAAAA) and the National Association of State
Units on Aging (NASUA). These are supplemented by the efforts
of the National Association of Nutrition Directors, the National
Institute of Senior Centers, the nationally based mass membership
organizations, and the new ad hoc coalitions on aging. Repeating
the question, "Decentralization to whom," I find it is not to older
persons. It is not to the community. It is not to the public at large.
Rather, it is to members of the aging network structure, which is
comprised of bureaucratic units and the trade associations mentioned earlier.

Now to the question, "Decentralization for what?" In implementing the Older Americans Act, the Administration on Aging
has increasingly been required to recognize trade associations as
legitimate representatives of the elderly. This recognition extends
far beyond NASUA and NAAAA or nutrition and senior center
programs. Partially in response to pressures from some membership organizations, former Commissioner on Aging Arthur Flemming fostered the organizational development of groups on aging,
many of which subsequently have become dominant organized interests that government, the public, and the aged must seriously
contend with. Older Americans Act demonstration project monies
were employed to support the development of these various trade
associations, much of whose activity within the aging network is
competitive. Unfortunately, however, as observed in Chapter Four,
interest-group policy making is not altogether democratic—contrary to pluralist mythology.

Current consequences have been the development and support of a network of agencies and their trade associations that feed
upon one another and upon federal policy makers and bureaucrats, seeking an ever-growing share of the resources available for
the aged in this country. It is the aged who become the "beneficiaries" of the scarcity that this network bartering inevitably pro-

duces (Binstock, 1972a). In gerontology the development of trade associations is consistent with the view that government should serve as the arbiter of the interests of private groups; it is consistent also with the creation of government policies designed to encourage the development of organized groups to advise the government.

The roots of this view of the government's role in relation to private groups are traced by Lowi to the Roosevelt administration and the National Recovery Administration (NRA), in which each industrial sector, service industry, and agricultural field was organized into committees of trade association representatives. To quote Lowi, "These representatives developed elaborate codes of fair competition . . . and . . . these codes became federal law" (1971, p. 75). Even though the NRA was declared unconstitutional because it permitted "excessive delegation of lawmaking power to private groups and government agencies," the practice of government regulation and control in cooperation with trade associations did not end with the Supreme Court's decision on the NRA; "it simply became somewhat less formal and explicit" (p. 75). The legitimation of trade associations and interest groups as appropriate participants in governmental affairs is also reflected in Galbraith's (1952) observation that support of countervailing power has become in modern times a major peacetime function of the federal government.

Government policy on aging similarly legitimates the role of organized groups, after initiating them in areas where they were supposedly needed. I share Lowi's concern that "the stamp of governmental legitimacy" on organized groups tends to "blind the American citizen to the real extent to which life is being controlled irresponsibly" (1971, p. 76). This lack of understanding contributes to the acceptance of trade associations as just another type of interest group and to the belief that policies resulting from interest-group pressures are democratic and fair. The official status accorded trade associations and other organizations representing important provider constituencies prevents their darker side from being seen. The public remains unaware of the control that these organizations exert over their members and the degree of power they have in legitimating and augmenting the work and careers of their members.

Decentralization is supposed to foster the participation of citizens in decisions affecting their lives. But under the Older Americans Act, public participation occurs *after* policy on the critical causes and solutions of problems has already been made. Dominant economic and political interests are not likely to be challenged by aging policies that are created and then variously and inconsistently implemented through decentralization mechanisms. Both the increasing number of policy decisions made by administering agencies and the heightened intensity of interest-group politics tend to minimize the influence of political leaders on public expenditures and priorities. As political decisions increasingly become administrative questions, the ability of legislatures to control budget priorities is reduced. (This loss of legislative initiative and power to the executive branch and to private economic interests is a trend noted some time ago by Mills. See *The Power Elite,* 1956.) Inevitably, the policies determined through private negotiation will be less liberal and less in the public interest than the legislative and electoral politics that they replace.

Similar considerations led Alford and Friedland to conclude that the U.S. government is bureaucratically structured in ways that protect dominant interests from political challenge; that is, its political fragmentation neutralizes nondominant interests and supports fiscal and policy dependence upon private economic power—thereby impeding legislative or electoral control over the structure of expenditures and revenues (1975, p. 473). In discussing the continued dependence of governments on private economic power, they point out that there are forms of taxation in which "fiscal capacity of all units of government is contingent upon the locational production and investment decisions of increasingly concentrated corporations" (p. 447). The relocation flexibility and financial resources of these businesses are constraints imposed by private business against tax raises that might drive them to seek other locations with better tax advantages. In this way local taxing systems are insulated from electoral challenge while being vulnerable to economic restraints imposed by private capital. Alford and Friedland sum up the problem: "As long as state revenues depend on taxes the autonomy of the state is limited by the necessity to avoid any policies that impact upon capital accumulation and growth"

(p. 448). One need mention only the example of New York City, where privately owned banks and financial institutions control critical state and municipal securities.

Decentralization is generally lauded for fairness because it supposedly assures pluralistic political participation. Since, however, it actually converts the democratic process into a process of bargaining among collectively organized interests, assumptions about fairness and equal opportunities must be questioned. Under many new federalism programs, one result of decentralization is that new special districts and jurisdictions have been created—for example, planning and service areas for area agencies on aging and planning districts for health systems agencies. These necessarily cause jurisdictional disputes and domain conflicts. More importantly, these entities often cross multiple geopolitical units for which there is no single electorate or other means of redress. Thus, decentralization not only allows public policy to be formed by a partnership of nonelected local administrators and private agencies, but it also reduces political (electoral) accountability for policy makers. Warren (1973a) contends that the creation of special authorities under decentralization results in a form of *centralization* because local authorities gain more power when program choices and implementation move into relatively protected bureaucratic and administrative arenas.

Under new federalism, decentralization reflects and strengthens the influence of what Beer (1976) calls "the professional bureaucratic complex" (the result of functional specialization) and "the intergovernmental lobby" (the result of territorial specialization). "The action and interaction" of these two types of influences constitute a new form of "representational federalism" that reflects the rise "within government itself" of "powerful new centers of influence on what government does" (Beer, 1978, p. 17). In his presidential address to the American Political Science Association, Beer remarked: "How rarely additions to the public sector have been initiated by the demands of voters or the advocacy of pressure groups or the platforms of political parties. On the contrary in the field of health, housing, transportation . . . it has been, in very great measure, people in government service, or closely associated with it, acting on the basis of their specialized and technical knowledge, who first perceived the problem, conceived the program, initially urged it on the president and Congress, went on to . . . lobby it through . . . and then saw to its administration" (1978, p. 17). Beer argues that the activity of these professionals and technocrats has been accompanied by demands of the intergovernmental lobby for fewer federal strings or more federal money. While the outcomes are mixed in terms of the centralizing and decentralizing tendencies of resulting policies, the essential question concerning each of these two new and powerful centers of influence is: Whom do they represent? Beer concludes by saying that he is uneasy about these "dilutions of the popular will [because] . . . the new structures have a strong connotation of corporate rather than personal representation" (1978, p. 20).

A reexamination of the assumption that increased local autonomy enhances responsiveness of leaders to the needs of citizens is critical, inasmuch as public participation in current decentralized new federalism policies is largely symbolic. In addition, comparative research on the relation of local autonomy to the willingness of officials to support efforts at social change indicates little association between these variables. Nor does community autonomy, defined as the opportunity for local institutions to take action on community needs and problems, appear to increase the involvement of the public in community affairs. These findings, based on cross-national research involving communities in the United States, Poland, India, and Yugoslavia, led the researchers to ask whether local autonomy did not actually provide "a closed preserve for leaders only" and then to observe: "Maybe the leaders themselves have broken the chain [of responsibility]; enjoying the fruits of autonomy in the exercise of greater personal influence, many are simply not inclined to pass on to others opportunities to participate more [and] many were . . . skeptical of such participation, feeling that decisions should be left to experts [or to] a few trusted and competent leaders. Thus, local elites stand close guard to prevent autonomy from going outside the gates of their own political power" (Jacob, 1975, p. 55).

When a legislative enactment sets few central directions or when its implementation and actual policies are worked out through a decentralized system of independent agencies, those who are well organized and well informed have a clear advantage over the general public. Although decentralization policies sometimes generate new agencies, the political establishment is usually affected only during the first round of organization: "Once new groups have been formed, they take on all the oligarchic trappings of previously organized groups, and the character of true representation in the society has hardly been affected at all. Thus, decentralization through delegation of power to lower levels almost always results in unequal access and group domination of the public situation" (Lowi, 1971, p. 78). In other words, decentralization is one mechanism for delegating critical program and policy decisions to progressively lower levels of authority; decisions then come to represent a combination of interest-group pressures and low-level bureaucratic processing.

Lowi argues that the only way out of the current crisis of legitimacy for public programs is "not to yield [policies and their implementation] directly to private claims, but quite independently to determine the control over them through clear laws that do not depend on the good wishes or the participatory practices of any of the subjects of these laws. If such laws were for a time properly and vigorously administered by duly constituted governmental administrative bodies . . . one might at some point . . . anticipate a proper and effective decentralization. . . . Until such time as true federal power and a clear national commitment to racial equality and economic equity have been established beyond a doubt, decentralization is abdication" (1971, p. 80).

Political and Economic Functions of Decentralization. A major consequence of decentralized national programs that affect the elderly—Title III of the Older Americans Act, Title XX of the Social Security Act, and general revenue sharing—is that they neutralize consumer and political mobilization by shifting the focal point for social action from a central, national locus to many local jurisdictions. This shift of focus has four results.

First, it weakens the capacity of all but the most well-organized, stable, and well-funded organizations to build and maintain momentum, for it becomes necessary to engage in multiple social action efforts across the nation; that is, to influence policy for the aged it becomes necessary to try to influence officials in some six hundred area agencies (or in fifty-eight thousand localities in the case of general revenue sharing). Further, within any single location for Older Americans Act programs, efforts must again be divided across the multiple townships, cities, and counties that comprise the artificially created substate boundaries of the planning and service areas for which the area agencies are assigned jurisdictional responsibility.

Second, it places human services demand on the most fiscally vulnerable government level of decision making—the local level. With decentralization, decisions about services for the disadvantaged are located precisely where pressures to control social expenses are greatest and necessarily the most conservative. The building and sustenance of the local economy requires local governments to minimize business taxation and to provide other economic incentives in order to prevent businesses from relocating to more economically favorable sites. The local economy may thus be seriously affected by private market considerations over which local officials have little control (except for their capacity to provide favorable fiscal treatment).

Third, it places human services decisions on the governmental level that is most accessible and most easily politicized. Local decisions about human services are much more open to public scrutiny, participation, and conflict than are national ones, and their fiscal effects are felt much more directly and immediately than are those of decisions made in Washington, D.C.

Fourth, because of the extreme variability in goal choices and implementation processes that decentralization allows, it is almost impossible to evaluate the results of programs. One might almost say that it will never be possible to assess the consequences of decentralization for the disadvantaged.

Because of these four factors, incrementalism in financing and budgeting is the most probable outcome of demands at the local level. Neither innovation nor structural change is likely under decentralized public policies, and the predominantly incremental funding patterns brought about by decentralized programs may well have various consequences. They may, for instance, prevent the restructuring of the local tax base, as well as of program and expenditure priorities. Again, the incremental approach "often prevents an immediate state response to current crises. . . . New programs often cut into the budgetary allocations or bureaucratic

authority of existent agencies and are therefore difficult to institute. On the one hand, a delayed state response may further pol-
iticize social groups [that] make new kinds of more expensive demands. On the other hand, the expanded operation of existent
ineffective programs is extremely costly" (Friedland, Alford, and
Piven, 1977, p. 27). It also happens that "fundamental conflicts
over . . . allocation . . . are transposed into marginal adjustments in
budgetary priorities. In the absence of sufficient legislative capacity
to radically restructure budgetary allocations and/or the organization of public finance, social groups [that] receive few benefits
from private accumulation or public expenditure have little incentive for political participation. The continuous flow of public expenditure for accumulation is reproduced and further entrenched
in the allocative routines of the state" (p. 23).

   Trade-offs. Specifically, what are some of the potential trade-
offs involved in the decentralization policies of the Older Americans Act? In Chapter Seven, I discuss issues of accountability and
decentralization, including Warren's (1973b) notion of the trade-
offs that occur when uniform standards and national goals are
abandoned. Issues of national priorities and central program
goals are among the most significant in understanding the consequences of public policy determination by decentralized processes. Trade-offs under the Older Americans Act illustrate some
of the major questions that decentralized public policies raise. For
example, how much state and local commitment to long-term
planning and coherent service strategies can we realistically expect
in the face of the growing fiscal constraints and intensified local
political pressures that occur when decision making and resource
allocations are brought closer to home? How likely are program
and allocation decisions to be politically motivated rather than
need-based under such conditions? How compatible is decentralization with rational planning if it results in the replacement of
national goals by the diversified outcomes of local political maneuvering?

   When priorities derived from planning conflict with expressed citizen preferences, the trade-off in implementation has
been to create symbolic participatory roles for older consumers so
that the planner's reality receives institutional legitimation without
threat of significant interference from the supposed beneficiaries.

This has been one result of the ambiguous mandates of the Older Americans Act. Further, what can rational planning at the local level be expected to accomplish in the face of growing awareness that "the root problems of the modern metropolis are not technical but political, and . . . expertise is largely irrelevant to the situation" (Thernstrom, 1969)? Yet, the continued imposition of rational planning strategies, along with the continuing hope that area agencies will successfully develop coordinated, comprehensive service systems in geographical areas over which agency planners have little authority, is part of an ideology whose support apparently does not depend on its ability to ameliorate social problems (Warren, 1973a; Estes, 1974b).

One of the potentially most serious results of the devolution of authority for program direction and emphasis under the Older Americans Act is the possible diminution or relinquishing of national goals. This may result either through state and local discretionary variations in implementation or as a consequence of diminished congressional oversight, which some have argued results from new federalism strategies. Decentralization under the Older Americans Act, with its characteristic ambiguity, tends to produce extreme fragmentation in problem-solving approaches nationwide, which in turn has weakened the impact of programs on both the personal lives of the aged and their aggregate social condition.

How compatible is the state and area agency discretion permitted under the Older Americans Act with the application of national performance standards? As described earlier, the performance reporting system begs the question by asking area agencies to set their own performance standards, which are first aggregated at the state level and then aggregated again for national performance reports. Questions already raised are: Who is accountable to whom and for what in a national program that permits self-evaluation of performance and refuses to set uniform standards? Can national goals be realized when there is such wide variability in state and local performance expectations? And unless we resolve the dilemma of accountability and decentralization, how can we know the effects of our national policies? Finally, what, if anything, do we know about citizen preferences as they influence policies for the aged?

IX

Citizen Participation of the Aged in Policy and Program Implementation

The true debate is not about participation but control [Bailey, 1975, p. 39].

Citizen participation has long been considered one of the keystones of American democracy. Public school boards, local governments, and political parties with their roots in local organization, as well as innumerable voluntary associations, have traditionally provided the means for citizen participation. To counter the more recent development of powerful interest-group lobbies, public interest lobbies such as Common Cause were established in the late 1960s and early 1970s; many of them, however, focused on their own special interest—children's television, nutrition, the environment, and so forth. Few developed the kind of grass roots citizen involvement that characterized Common Cause or such powerful special interest lobbies as the Chamber of Commerce.

Note: The author gratefully acknowledges the assistance of Betsy Robinson in the initial review and analysis of the literature relevant to this chapter.

Since the early 1960s government policy has encouraged citizen participation in federal programs, using approaches that range from the Poverty Program's mandated involvement of the poor in decision making to the advisory roles permitted the elderly under the Older Americans Act. The elderly and their advocates have chosen a variety of different channels, including those provided by the Older Americans Act, in an effort to influence public policy. Following the tradition of pluralism and interest-group policy, the elderly have formed several national special interest organizations, some with state and local affiliates, to organize, advocate, and lobby on their behalf. Some of the elderly have taken part in the activities of the major political parties as a means to influence in public policy on aging, as well as in policies that might promote the general welfare. Others have taken advantage of the opportunity to participate in the state and area agency advisory councils and the nutrition project advisory committees mandated by the Older Americans Act. Another course of action has been to work at the federal level in such special interest areas as health, income, education, employment, and welfare in an effort to bring about a more equitable distribution of wealth. But how effective have these efforts been? What influence do the elderly have on policies and programs that affect them directly? Do the elderly need to reexamine the present avenues of citizen participation and consider a more activist approach? This chapter will examine the role of citizen participation in the implementation of several important federal programs—the Older Americans Act, as well as general and special revenue sharing programs.

Power and Participation

Legislative enactments and government policies set forth the appropriate degrees of formal and discretionary power to be assigned to those who design and implement policies. These prescriptions about who has power in particular areas of policy may actually reduce the need for the participation of some groups while increasing the need for participation by others.

The fact that participatory roles are provided for citizens does not automatically mean that those citizens have power. On the contrary! Alford and Friedland (1975) make an important distinction between three categories of participatory power: (1) participation without power (symbolic power); (2) participation with power; and (3) power without participation (systemic or structural power). Participation without power, or symbolic power, results in the siphoning off of potential political leadership into ineffective channels of influence, preventing challenge to the dominant institutions of society. An example of participation without power is the purely advisory role that limits one to reacting or responding to the initiatives, plans, and decisions of others. Although the Older Americans Act and new federalism programs theoretically provide participatory opportunities for the elderly, these opportunities are largely symbolic because of their advisory nature. The interests of the administering agencies are built into all these programs because they hold policy making authority. Public participation under the Older Americans Act is structured so that it functions as a "repressed interest" (Alford, 1976). Elderly citizens have built-in disadvantages when it comes to determining the policies and outcomes of programs that are supposed to benefit them.

Regulated industries provide an example of power with participation. Through special access to officials (at regulatory agencies, for example) and involvement in the creation of special agencies, they are able to limit and shape the jurisdictions of regulatory bodies. Similar forms of power with participation are the inclusion of trade association representatives of state and area agencies on aging in informal advisory sessions to the commissioner on aging during formulative and implementation stages of a policy that may affect their interests. Administration on Aging review committees for research and demonstration grants also include such representation. Often a means of special interest protection, such review and regulatory and other ad hoc and informal mechanisms of access limited to relatively few interest groups ensure that their views are heard; they insulate their interests (whether popular or not) from political challenge.

Power without participation is exemplified when private groups make decisions about capital investments that are then adopted by government. In this way many public expenditures come to be controlled by the private rather than the public sector. Under these conditions of low political visibility, economic power can be exercised with maximum freedom. An example is provided by the billions of dollars currently flowing into private and community hospitals for expansion or renovation at a time when hospital beds are almost everywhere in excess supply and the federal government is attempting to curb new construction and expensive renovations. These added costs are then met through increased per diem charges that are paid for by third parties, including Medicare, Medicaid, and private health insurance. State laws designed to regulate such construction usually provide grandfather clauses that exempt most or all of the funds currently in the pipeline. Local health planning agencies are usually helpless to stop new construction because it has the support of powerful local interest groups, including the hospital in question, physicians, banks, and the construction industry.

One of the most pervasive forms of power without participation is found in the legitimation of the expert's definition. Problem definitions that are supposedly objective, neutral, and nonpolitical provide support for the perspectives of those who are defining the issue—usually elites. Decisions that are seen as requiring professional or technical judgments simultaneously justify the exclusion of laypersons—who are defined as inexpert and incompetent—from meaningful participation. These definitional processes promote public acquiescence; the layperson's intelligence and experience are systematically devalued, and a definitional vacuum is created into which professionals and other organized interests may move.

In addition, the public has been "socialized from infancy to believe it is incompetent to deal with important decisions because they are technical and complex; [therefore, it] is . . . satisfied with ritualistic participation that stays within the limits set by professional and governmental authorities and which serves chiefly to induce conformity" (Edelman, 1977, p. 126). As a consequence, those most seriously affected by a problem are most likely to be routinely excluded from the process by which problem and solution are defined.

What is perhaps most important about participation without power is that the provision of even nominal, symbolic roles fosters the illusion that policies and programs are democratically made and implemented. Such perceptions, in turn, restrain or moderate the demand for more meaningful citizen power. Also, problems raised by citizen participants are explained away as minor misunderstandings or small differences in preference. The positive association of participation with the mystique of democracy permits the management and containment of citizen input by agency leaders. "Such routines perpetuate and legitimate existing inequalities and influence" (Edelman, 1977, p. 126). The purportedly democratic basis of politics and programs masks the inequalities that underlie their minimal achievements and diverts attention away from the relationship of the policy or program to the severe deprivation suffered by target groups. When individuals with little social status are given even very limited participatory roles, they are still discouraged from resisting policies. But their very participation minimizes the likelihood that these persons will be perceived as unfairly treated. Mandates for citizen participation, particularly advisory participation, that have no authority and no legal standing outside of the organization to be advised constitute a way of mollifying target groups. Citizens who so advise are likely to adopt dominant organizational perspectives, resulting in a net loss of their political resources. Political power for the disadvantaged ultimately resides in their potential for collective action. Symbolic participation in citizen advisory councils diminishes the possibility of collective action, reducing the primary source of power available to the disadvantaged. Thus, as potential leaders are drawn into routine administrative thickets, their energies and capacities are rechanneled, and the likelihood of their organizing constituencies diminishes.

Citizen Participation in Federal Social Programs

VanTil and VanTil's study (1970) documents a shift in the citizen participation requirements of government programs. The study concludes that following the citizen activism of the early 1960s, we are now returning to the traditional citizen participation mode in which elites and nonelites join in minimal advisory activities. This observation is particularly applicable to the general and special revenue sharing programs enacted in the mid 1970s. Though these laws consistently employ language providing for public participation, many of the provisions are for roles even more perfunctory than advisory ones. For example, prior to the 1976 Amendments to the Older American Act, a variety of non-required citizen participation mechanisms had been employed by cities and counties receiving funds from general revenue sharing, ranging from advisory committees to survey opinion polls regarding the allocation of funds. A survey for the National Science Foundation found that 59 percent of cities over three hundred thousand and 76.2 percent of cities between one and three hundred thousand had established advisory committees (though not specifically for general revenue sharing) to advise on budget or financial matters. The National Clearinghouse on Revenue Sharing, however, issued a highly critical report on the use of advisory groups, stating that "citizen advisory groups, even where they exist, have little real power. Their function may be to make recommendations for allocating a limited amount of money among many claimants—thus relieving public officials of the political burden inherent in such decision making" (National Science Foundation, 1975, p. 59).

Of all the means used by the major revenue-sharing programs to encourage citizen participation (see Table 8), public hearings are the most common. Although it is widely acknowledged that "effective citizen participation requires more than the passive dissemination of information" (National Science Foundation, 1975, p. 58), many states and localities have regarded this provision as being met simply by publication of the planned and/or actual-use reports in the newspaper.

As the keystone of new federalism, the General Revenue Sharing (GRS) program was heralded by the Nixon administration as an important step toward government decentralization. Nevertheless, experience to date suggests that the "program has not decidedly changed the nature and type of participation in the political processes of recipient governments" (Nathan, Adams, and Associates, 1977, p. 164). Studies of the scope and extent of citizen participation in the decision-making process of GRS reached similar negative conclusions (Waldhorn and others, 1975; Lovell, Korey, and Weber, 1975; Nathan, Manvel, and Calkins, 1975; Rondinelli, 1975). The General Accounting Office (GAO) findings have been succinctly summarized as follows: "GAO found that only one third

Table 8. Participation Requirements in Major Revenue-Sharing Programs Affecting the Aged

Revenue-Sharing Program	Planned Use or Plan Published	Citizen Input into Planning Process	Formal Citizen Participation Mechanism	Public Hearings and Meetings	Actual-Use Report Published	Environmental Impact Report
General-revenue sharing				X	X	
Title XX (social services)	X			X		
Community development (housing)	X	X		X		X
Comprehensive Employment and Training Act			X	X		
Urban Mass Transportation Act				X		X

Source: Zucker and Estes, 1976, p. 42.

of the 240 cities and counties surveyed indicated increased citizen participation in the planning of local revenue-sharing allocations over normal public involvement in regular budgetary processes. The remaining two thirds claimed that the program had not affected citizen participation" (Rondinelli, 1975, p. 330). After initial broad interest in the general revenue sharing program, public interest subsided. Juster observes that "overall group participation in hearings appears to have been limited to organizations already in existence prior to GRS" (1976, p. 11).

Although citizen participation was not the chief purpose of the GRS program, federal and other officials and others have claimed that revenue-sharing programs provide a means of increasing such participation, particularly at the local level. A key feature of the State and Local Assistance Act amendments of 1976 was the strengthening of the public participation provisions. Under the 1976 amendments recipient governments are required to hold two separate hearings prior to the appropriation of revenue-sharing funds. As described by the Office of Revenue Sharing: "Each hearing requires ten (10) days public notice prior to the hearing date, and may be held in conjunction with other governmental meetings or budget proceedings. Legal notices are not required, but there are specific requirements for the content of each notice. Recipient governments are expected to make a special effort to involve senior citizens, and to notify all news media of the hearings (including minority, bilingual, and foreign language media). If governments are not required to adopt a budget in accordance with state and/or local law, they must hold the required hearings before appropriating or spending any of their revenue-sharing funds" (U.S. Department of the Treasury, 1978, p. 1). Senior citizen organizations were to be allowed to make their views heard while the budget was still in the planning stage: "Special care should be given to notification prior to the hearings; notices may be posted at senior citizen centers and other locations frequented by senior citizens and should be mailed to organizations representing these citizens for their use in advising their members" (1978, p. 2).

In the early stages of revenue sharing when there was a greater degree of citizen participation, procedures were employed that gave the program visibility in communities and encouraged citizen and group participation in decisions about uses for GRS funds. The 1976 amendments of the revenue-sharing act would also speak to citizen participation through public hearings. But how meaningful participatory opportunities actually are depends on the politics of the budgetary process. A major point here is whether revenue-sharing funds are treated separately or are merged into the regular budgetary process.

Current political theories which argue that standard budgetary procedures act as constraints upon meaningful citizen input appear substantiated by the two major studies of revenue sharing. According to Juster, "When GRS is handled just like other local funds with no special hearings or committees, opportunities for citizen participation should be less common" (1976, p. 175). Significant findings related to citizen participation, budgetary procedures, and the fiscal position of state and local governments have also been reported by Nathan, Adams, and Associates. Although the data from their two rounds of field observation cover the period prior to the 1976 amendments, they highlight a major constraint upon opportunities for citizen involvement: "Twenty-seven jurisdictions were reported to have completely merged revenue-sharing funds into their regular budgets during the second round of field observations. Six of the eight state governments were classified as merged, as were approximately one half of the city governments in the sample. More than one half of the city governments with over 100,000 population were classified as merged, compared to approximately one quarter of those under 100,000. A distinct relationship was also observed between fiscal pressure and the decision to merge shared revenue. Two thirds of the local governments characterized as under moderate or extreme fiscal pressure during the second round were included in the merged category, compared to only one fifth of the localities under light or no fiscal pressure" (Nathan, Adams, and Associates, 1977, p. 111). An examination of the budget procedures of recipient governments for fiscal year 1974 led to the conclusion that "the probability of revenue sharing playing a prominent role in the budget and being afforded some type of special treatment is significantly reduced as the overall fiscal health of a recipient juris-diction deteriorated (p. 114).

These findings are confirmed by Juster, who summarizes the current relation between citizen participation and local fiscal processes as follows: "Over time, whatever special treatment was initially given to revenue-sharing funds declined as they were in-corporated into the regular budgetary process. Fewer cities of all sizes held special hearings on revenue sharing the second year than the first. Furthermore, local officials overwhelmingly expressed their opposition to requiring the formation of citizen advisory com-mittees as a condition of the revenue-sharing program" (1976, p. 165).

Case study data reported by the National Clearinghouse on Revenue Sharing also emphasized the limited value of public hear-ings on revenue sharing when they are held as part of the regular budget process (National Science Foundation, 1975). In San Fran-cisco, for example, there have been no public hearings specifically devoted to GRS allocations since Mayor Joseph Alioto left office in January 1976. Rather than risk the fanfare of separate and highly visible public hearings, the mayor's office considered the requirement to hold planned-use hearings fulfilled by merging GRS budget issues with the general city and county budget hear-ings. GRS allocations to San Francisco for the fiscal year 1978–1979 illustrate the outcome in expenditure areas: $7.3 million for fire services; $5.7 million for police; $4.15 million for recreation; and $5.2 million for municipal transportation. Thus, (sub)merging revenue-sharing funds into the regular budget process means less visibility for the program and even less opportunity for citizen par-ticipation as to the use of funds.

Juster's study (1976) revealed that cities that held initial hearings and/or established formal mechanisms for citizen partic-ipation spent a greater proportion of their revenue-sharing funds on social services. These findings were confirmed by the General Accounting Office, which "found that most increased participa-tion, where it did take place, resulted from interest-group activities to influence allocation of revenue-sharing funds for special pro-grams" (National Science Foundation, 1975, p. 63). In the same vein, Waldhorn found (1975) that those cities that scored highest in citizen participation factors also scored highest in outcome factors. This suggests that increased levels of citizen participation do have significant effect on local outcomes.

The 1975 Social Security amendments (Public Law 93–647), which created a new Title XX, marked a further shift in decision-making authority from the federal to the state level. The removal of mandated services for certain categories of recipients in the 1975 legislation was supposed to permit more responsive state priority setting. The amendments gave states the general mandate to include one service directed to each of the Title XX goals and at least three services for recipients of Supplementary Security Income. Because states are free under Title XX to select services that meet particular needs of their own residents, substantial shifts can occur in the distribution of resources among specific subgroups of the broadly eligible population. The current fluidity of what was previously a share-specified and categorical program makes access to channels of influence almost imperative for disadvantaged groups seeking their share of social services in the state.

This raises the questions of what mechanisms exist for public participation in the process by which priorities for needs, services, and population groups are determined by each state; what roles (actual and potential) there are for the aged; and what influence these participatory processes have on Title XX programs. The public participation requirements under Title XX are as follows:

> 1. Ninety days prior to the beginning of the state's service year . . . [it] publishes and makes generally available . . . to the public a proposed comprehensive annual services program plan prepared by the agency [Sec. 2004 (2)].
>
> 2. Public comment on the proposed plan is accepted for a period of at least forty-five days [Sec. 2004 (03)].
>
> 3. At least forty-five days after publication of the proposed plan and prior to the beginning of the state's services program year . . . [it] publishes a final comprehensive annual services program prepared by the agency designed pursuant to the requirements of Section 2003 (d) (1) (c) [Sec. 2004 (4)].

"A Citizen's Handbook" on program options and public participation under Title XX of the Social Security Act (1975) boasts that there are new opportunities for citizens: "Title XX puts it up to states and their citizens to make their social services programs fit the needs of people in local communities as effectively as possible. Until now every state's social services plan has had to be approved by the federal government. Under Title XX the content of a state's services plan will be subject to review by the state's citizens rather than to approval by the federal government. To assure that citizens have an opportunity to review the state services plan, the law requires an open planning process. This includes a public review and comment period of at least forty-five days" ("Social Services '75," 1975, p. 3). The role of citizen organizations in planning is described as follows: "Individuals and organizations can help by giving state and local agencies as much information as possible about community needs and resources. . . . Such help can be given by writing letters, participating in any public hearings on social services, and joining citizen groups actively interested in social services program development" (1975, p. 15). Opportunities for the aged to influence Title XX priorities are no different from those for the average citizen—in other words, they are minimal; there are no provisions for direct citizen contact with those who set program policies.

The growth of many private grass roots organizations at the local level has accompanied the continued decentralization of national social programs. Most striking is the diversity in type and scope of these organizations as well as the variety of issues to which they attend (Perlman, 1976). The growing antigovernment sentiment represented in recent taxpayer revolts—for example, California's successful 1978 property tax initiative (Jarvis-Gann)—typifies what Perlman (1976) describes as a trend toward local self-reliance. Perlman argues that the shift is from national to neighborhood issues. To the extent that these trends continue, the power potential of the aged may be diminished because their interest group efforts have been primarily successful in national level efforts. Further, the major issues that affect the aged are national, not neighborhood, ones. Where else can policies on social security, retirement, income maintenance, or national health insurance be settled but at the federal level? And the kind of negligible public participation now observable in new federalism programs will do little to create national level concern or to influence public policies of direct benefit to the aged.

Unfortunately, the negative consequence of decentralization is greatest for weakly organized and unorganized interests. The increasing discretionary authority provided states and localities under both revenue sharing and the Older Americans Act permits broad latitude in altering or eliminating services and eligible classes of participants. This autonomy for administering agencies makes it possible for certain population groups to be shortchanged in ways that the earlier more centralized, standardized, and specified procedures did not permit. The variability, ambiguity, and complexity of new federalism programs necessitate systematically organized efforts by older persons and their advocates to ensure influence on policy decisions.

Little information is available about the participation of the aged in Title XX planning; nevertheless, data on public participation in the Title XX program are not reassuring. While Rose, Zorn, and Radin's study of twenty-three states shows that all twenty-three were complying with the minimal regulatory mandates for public participation and that eighteen exceeded these requirements, they admit that "anything more than after-the-fact public involvement will only occur at the option of individual states" (1976, p. 26). Additional public involvement opportunities provided by states took the form of advisory committees, hearings, and questionnaire surveys. The optimism of the authors cannot cover up two facts of major importance: (1) states may do very little to involve the public if they so choose, and (2) the forms of participation states have chosen are essentially reactive involvement modes rather than action modes in which citizens define their own needs and priorities. This conclusion is substantiated by United Way of America's assessment project (Tokarz, 1977), which reported that almost nothing was done to solicit data on preferences or needs from consumers. Similarly, an Urban Institute report states that "a significant degree of the negative elements of the Title XX process identified . . . relate to the lack of public participation or its absence of effect on the resource allocation decision-making process, particularly during the second year of Title XX implementation. The findings in the fifty-one jurisdiction survey also support the contention that lack of external influence limited the degree of service allocation changes or focused it in particular directions" (Feild, Millar, and Benton, 1978, p. 15). Tokarz (1977) argues that Title XX is so complicated that most citizens cannot understand it; this undoubtedly has minimized citizen participation in the program. Following the consistent trend away from Poverty Program efforts to establish paragovernments of policy-making citizens toward the more diluted policy influence of citizens in the Model Cities Program (through the imposition of planning mandates that inserted professionals in the decision-making process), the Older Americans Act took one more step toward limiting citizen influence. Older Americans Act provisions for involvement of the aged as "advisers" are consistent with the more limited role that revenue-sharing programs accord citizen input. As noted, with revenue sharing such input is almost entirely a matter of hearings, with decision making firmly located and insulated within the relevant government units.

At the federal level, the Older Americans Act created two formal means for citizen participation in the development of national policies—the Federal Council on Aging and the White House Conference on Aging. The 1973 amendments to the Older Americans Act created a fifteen-member advisory council—the Federal Council on Aging—to advise and assist the president, the secretary of Health, Education, and Welfare, the commissioner on aging, and Congress. The council's duties are to: (1) review and evaluate on a continuing basis federal policies for the aging; (2) make recommendations to the president, the secretary, the commissioner, and Congress about federal policies on the aging and federally conducted or assisted programs related to or affecting them; (3) inform the public about the problems and needs of the aging by collecting and disseminating information, conducting or commissioning studies, and issuing publications and reports; and (4) provide public forums for discussing and publicizing the problems and needs of the aging (Federal Council on the Aging, 1978). Council members are presidential appointees confirmed by the Senate. Ten members of the council are themselves older persons, although they and the other members are by law supposed to represent national organizations with an interest in the elderly, business, labor, and the general public. The principle of interest-group advising is thus institutionalized by means of the council.

Another means of public participation in the development of national policies is the White House Conference on Aging. Recent analysis of three decades of such conferences leads Pratt to conclude that they "may be a means of 'cooling out' malcontents by appearing to deal with their problems" (Pratt, 1978, p. 72). But the influence of a number of private groups was solidified during events surrounding the 1971 White House Conference on Aging. Following their exclusion from the planning process for the 1971 Conference, several nationally based senior citizen groups publicly expressed their outrage during hearings before the Senate Special Committee on Aging in the spring of 1971. After the groups engaged in a series of threats of boycotts and spoke of convening a "Black House Conference on Aging," President Nixon appointed former Health, Education, and Welfare Secretary Arthur Flemming as conference chairman "to get things back on the track." As a result of the meetings that Flemming held with leaders of six protesting groups, the number of delegates to the conference was increased and a task force was created to monitor conference planning; organized senior citizen groups were assigned a specified number of slots for delegates and task-force members. In addition, the chairman agreed to a formal statement, prepared by these organizations, which he subsequently read (Pratt, 1978).

Thus, by the early 1970s, national policy on aging was beginning to emerge as a partnership between public officials and organized groups from the private sector. The 1973 comprehensive services amendments to the Older Americans Act significantly expanded the number of organizations in the field, and the aging network now exceeds thirty-five hundred agencies and organizations. The question is, to what extent do these aging organizations represent the elderly, and particularly the most disadvantaged of the elderly?

Between 1965 and 1973 state units on aging were required to receive advisory assistance from consumers organized into advisory councils. The state unit and area agency advisory bodies created in 1973 were instituted to provide consumer input for state and area plans, respectively. State and project level nutrition advisory bodies also were legislatively mandated in 1972. Participation of the elderly in public hearings and state plan review and comment procedures under the Older Americans Act nevertheless appears minimal and symbolic. After studying state units in fifteen states, Applied Management Sciences (1975) concluded that state unit planning made use of very little outside input. Even input from other agencies was found to be extremely limited, with only two or three of the state units reporting such participation. Applied Management Sciences also noted that none of the state units interviewed changed the final drafts of their state plans as a result of testimony in public hearings, despite the fact that the public hearing is supposedly a primary planning tool. In addition, "Chairpersons of at least two state advisory committees also indicated that the [Fiscal Year 1975] public hearing did not reflect the true needs of the older consumer because the hearings in their respective states were structured to exclude older consumers most in need. . . . only three [of fifteen state unit] directors stated that the public hearings were useful as a needs assessment technique" (Applied Management Sciences, 1975, p. 518).

Under the Older Americans Act, the role of older persons is not one of creating radical, broad-scale, institutional changes, because the act essentially sets forth a planning and services strategy whose object is to develop and coordinate comprehensive service systems. The Older Americans Act is not designed to provide income transfers, to redistribute power resources to older persons, to develop leadership, or to organize the elderly as a constituency to act in their own behalf. Advocacy is left to state units and area agencies, and even their exercise of this function is not clearly spelled out (O'Brien and Wetle, 1975). In sum, the functions that citizen advisers can exercise under the Older Americans Act are severely restricted, especially in view of the narrow interpretation given by the Administration on Aging to Section 903.50 (c) of Federal Regulations on Advisory Assistance under Title III (*Federal Register,* 1973). According to the Administration on Aging, the primary purpose of the advisory committee is "to serve as an ongoing means by which the views of older consumers of services, service providers, and others in the field of aging are taken into account. . . . The regulations do not assign policy or decision-making functions to the committee. Authority to establish policies and make final decisions governing the conduct of the Title III and VII programs is vested in the state agency" (Administration on Aging, 1976a, p. 2).

Since 1973, efforts of state and area agencies to expand the limited participatory role of elders beyond advice giving have been systematically thwarted. The interpretation of federal regulations on advisory assistance has been that advisory councils are limited to advisory activities, even in those rare instances when a governor or mayor chooses to strengthen the participation of the aged. For example, in 1975, one governor granted a council of older persons a policy-making role by executive order. He was prohibited from carrying out this order by the Administration on Aging's refusal to approve the state's annual plan for aging until it rectified this "error."

Further, the Administration on Aging discourages citizen involvement in state and area agencies that are organized around decision-making commissions by arguing that "such commission[s] will not satisfy requirements of Section 903.50 (c). All state agencies on aging, no matter how they may be constituted, must have the benefit of advice and assistance from an independent advisory body" (Administration on Aging, 1976b). Because it is too costly for most agencies to run two councils simultaneously (a policy commission and an advisory committee), the incentive is for state and area agencies to abolish their policy-making commissions, since they are discretionary, in favor of the mandatory advisory body. Federal regulations do not specifically prohibit policy-making roles for advisory councils; it is simply that Administration on Aging issuances interpret them as doing this. An alternative interpretation of Section 903.50 (c) could just as well be that advisory assistance represented the minimum form of activity and that a more direct (policy-making) involvement for advisory committees was a discretionary decision of state and area agencies.

Advice Without Influence

Advising, then, is the major type of participation prescribed for the aged under the Older Americans Act. In situations in which the power of citizen participants is relatively low, advisory body representatives are likely to serve one or more of the following functions for the state or area agencies: (1) legitimation of the organization's or planner's efforts (Kaplan, 1970); (2) sharing in the public symbols of authority and public responsibility without the transfer of substantive power (Selznick, 1949); (3) advocating expansion of the organization's or planner's programs by petitioning for resources at state or local levels (Mogulof, 1970); and/or (4) shielding the organization's or planner's decisions from opposition and criticism (Lauffer, 1974). Such functions are typified by what Selznick (1949) has defined as "formal co-optation." *Co-optation* is "the process of absorbing new elements into the organization. . . . The use of formal co-optation . . . does not envision the transfer of actual power. The forms of participation are emphasized but action is channeled so as to fulfill the administrative functions while preserving the locus of significant decision in the hands of the initiating group" (Selznick, 1949, pp. 13–14).

In Older Americans Act programs the aged are confined to citizen involvement rather than citizen action roles. As defined by Warren, Rose, and Bergunder (1974), citizen involvement roles provide for "appropriate input" from the client population but are predicated on the acceptance of the agency's viability and rationale, with citizen input supporting and bolstering that viability and rationale. It is a kind of involvement highly compatible with the organization's basic technical, administrative and institutional rationale. Assumptions are that the views of responsible citizens will be congruent with those of agency staff and that citizen participants will support agency programs, if only they receive sufficient education. Citizen involvement means "at the most education and at the least a pretense at consultation . . . [what education there is orients clients] toward professional views based on consensualism" (Bailey, 1975, p. 39).

While involvement roles focus on obtaining desired services, citizen action roles focus on obtaining political power in order to make the system responsible to participant-defined needs and demands. Underlying differences between involvement and action roles revolve around (1) who defines the problems and needs of the constituency, (2) what procedures are to be employed in making those definitions, and (3) how solutions to problems are to be implemented. There are perhaps seven critical factors that enhance or limit the influence of citizen participants and that are especially relevant to the Older Americans Act.

First, there is considerable ambiguity regarding the rights and responsibilities of older persons in advisory roles under provisions of the Older Americans Act. The issuances establishing the federal regulations on advisory participation under this act have consistently excluded advisers from policy-making roles. Policy roles are open to elders only if they become high-ranking employees of Older Americans Act programs. Such employment, however, has been minimal because of civil service and other age discrimination barriers—legislative language providing employment preference to the aged notwithstanding.

There are few guidelines regarding the responsibilities that older persons are to assume in their advisory capacities. Regulations specify only a review and comment role during the annual state and area planning sessions, both before and after public hearings. It is not specified whether such advice is to cover (or be limited to) administrative, bureaucratic, or technical questions or whether it is to include major policy considerations (for example, the direction of coordination/integration of a state's social service and nutrition projects), review and comment on grant applications, or other types of program development issues. Consistent with decentralization principles, state and area agencies are allowed to specify the roles and functions of their advisory committees, and agencies vary widely in their exercise of this option. The extent to which older persons are defined as appropriately involved in policy arenas reflects in large measure the degree of power that they will hold.

Still another participatory mechanism is the public hearing. But, although state and area plans are subject to public hearing and review by an advisory body, these processes are not likely to produce more than perfunctory citizen involvement. Perhaps most important, there is no requirement, and consequently little inducement, for a state or area agency to seriously consider the advice it receives through hearings and its advisory body. The inclination of any organization caught between an oversupply of requirements and an undersupply of resources is to minimize the time-consuming and tension-producing processes of obtaining input from extraorganizational leaders and advisers. And because of their limited roles, older citizen advisers are easily relegated to extraorganizational status.

The second dimension—ambiguity in the advisory/participation arena—relates to the criteria for membership in and the selection process for advisory boards. The Older Americans Act's agencies are asked to "take into account in connection with matters of general policy . . . the views of recipients of services under such plan" and to establish an advisory council consisting of "representatives of older individuals, local elected officials, and the general public" (Older Americans Act, 1978, p. 1523). But lack of specificity about the criteria for members and the process by which they are to be chosen allows for nondemocratic selection processes (or even "stacking" of an advisory group to exclude the disadvantaged, less powerful, more radical, or troublesome older persons). Also, the lack of clarity and specificity enables at least two different types of citizens to claim that they are representing older persons— those seriously disadvantaged in their old age and those participating in the social problems enterprise (for example, retired professionals), who do not identify themselves with the aged but instead speak for professional or organizational interests. The views of these different types of participants are likely to be markedly different, the former being more likely to represent a consumer perspective, and the latter the views of dominant social institutions, organizations, or professions. In addition, the federally regulated requirement of appointing advisory members who are "representatives of major public and private agencies and organizations" encourages the dilution of a consumer-oriented perspective on these boards, for it is just such coalition advisory structures that are characteristically dominated by their nonconsumer members (Mogulof, 1970).

Third, the character and attitude of the sponsoring organization is critical in determining the influence of older persons. As noted, the Administration on Aging has taken a dim view of giving policy authority to older persons. Thus, the legitimate, mandated federal advocate for older persons, the Administration on Aging, does not itself propose self-determination by the elderly even in Older Americans Act programs. Given this stand, it is hardly surprising that it is the exception rather than the rule for state units and area agencies to dignify with authority the advice or involvement of older persons. The elderly person is usually relegated to the role of client in Older Americans Act programs, and "interaction" for him or her comes down to cooperation. There is sufficient research to indicate that participants limited to cooperative roles are not likely to bring about program innovation or responsiveness (Warren, Rose, and Bergunder, 1974).

The age of an organization is also an important aspect of its character (Blumer, 1971). With regard to the Older Americans Act, community participants were usually not involved in the creation of the state or area agencies. Often, long before advisory bodies are formed, these agencies have developed regularized ways of doing things, solidifying the staff's vested interests (both formal and informal). In such instances, the entry of community participants is likely to be resisted, for they bring with them the threat that citizen power always poses to bureaucracies. Further, the more hierarchical and bureaucratic the organization, the less likely it is that advisory participants will be provided opportunities to create an impact on the unit. The orientation and commitment of key staff members of state and area agencies also are likely to play an important role in the type of citizen participation allowed and encouraged. It has been found, for example, that there is an inverse relationship between staff domination and citizen influence (Kaplan, 1970). In cases of staff domination, consumers function primarily to legitimize or sanction predetermined staff decisions.

Fourth, organizational inducements also determine the degree of citizen power. Under current conditions there is small reason for state or area agencies to involve older persons substantially in decision making. In addition to the Administration on Aging's negative position on consumer involvement, there has been little monitoring of state unit or area agency compliance with federal regulations on advisory assistance. For example, as late as July 1975, a program instruction was issued on this topic with reference to the state plan for fiscal year 1976, reminding state units of the requirement to establish advisory bodies. Since state level advisory bodies were a requirement even before the 1973 amendments, a logical question is, why has the mandate been enforced so loosely? This lack of accountability, one surmises, reflects the low salience of citizen advice in the Older Americans Act program. The lack of sanctions for dilatory action on compliance with advisory body regulations serves to encourage continued variability and minimal compliance in the implementation of Older Americans Act mandates requiring citizen participation. Even if organizational inducements existed for seriously involving older persons in decision making, opposition could be anticipated because of general organizational resistance to investing the required energy for utilizing and effectively benefiting from citizen input on program development and policy issues. Nothing short of major attitudinal or ideological commitments by key staff members can effectively provide the inducements essential to meaningful citizen participation.

The fifth factor associated with the degree of citizen involvement is the nature of target group. Poverty, despair, and skepticism about whether participation can make a difference are factors that minimize target group involvement in advisory activities. Further, according to the finding by O'Shea and Gray (1966) of a direct relationship between social class and participation, the poor tend to participate less than others. Fleisher and Kaplan (1978) also report the tendency for higher participation among those who perceive that their efforts make a difference. Without specified and enforced provisions for poor or minority representation, middle-class, retired professionals are most likely to be the consumers drawn into advisory capacities for aging programs.

The sixth factor affecting the influence of citizen participants is the extent to which they possess the skills requisite to leadership roles. More than charisma and organizational or verbal skills is required. For example, to participate effectively and contribute to policy decisions for the Older Americans Act, detailed knowledge of the regulations and of the policies and procedures for implementing the act is essential, not to mention having basic familiarity with the political realities of the environments in which the state units and area agencies operate. The Administration on Aging does not require state units or area agencies to provide training for their advisers. Nor is technical assistance regularly available to most advisory councils. If either occurs it is because of the foresight, beneficience, or faith of the state unit or area agency executives or their staffs—not because of some organizational or political necessity to provide these essential skills and resources.

Seventh, the extent to which there are tangible inducements for the target group to involve itself in programs meant to serve it is also important (Fleisher and Kaplan, 1978). There is usually, however, no financial remuneration that agencies for the elderly can provide their participants for expenses or time invested. Most advisory groups in these agencies have no staff or other resources to enable them to carry on their work. This, coupled with the aforementioned skepticism of many potential consumer participants, diminishes the incentive for those older persons who most need services to become involved in programs.

The most recent legislative enactments have not altered this situation. In the 1978 reauthorization deliberations there was virtually no consideration given to increasing the role of older persons by mandating the employment of elders in programs funded by the Older Americans Act or to augmenting the purely symbolic roles that older persons play as advisers in the act's programs. Despite the Age Discrimination Act and recent legislation extending the age for mandatory retirement, the issue of age discrimination in federal programs remains very much alive because of the structural pervasiveness of discriminatory practices, which vary in form across states and localities. The advisory functions of older persons in state and area planning and the nutrition program were untouched in the 1978 reauthorization. Similarly, the primarily advisory role of the Federal Council on Aging was left undisturbed in these recent amendments, although the council was given additional mandates for conducting selected studies such as analyzing "the numbers and incidence of low-income and minority participants in such programs" (Older Americans Act, 1978).

Thus, the major concerns of the aged appear to have had little influence on either the initial design or the subsequent amendments to the Older Americans Act. We have also seen that there are many barriers that prevent the elderly from playing a decision-making role in the programs and policies supposedly created for their benefit. These barriers, present in policy designs from the start, have been raised even higher by the various agencies charged with implementing programs for the elderly. Throughout this book I have examined these failings of the Older Americans Act and other federal policy initiatives for the aged in America. Now it is time to see if there are any solutions.

X

Social Policy
Alternatives: A
Redefinition of Problems,
Goals, and Strategies

━━━━━◘▱◘━━━━━◘▱◘━━━━━

A man's aging and his decline always takes place inside some given society: it is ultimately related to that society and to the place that the individual occupies within it [de Beauvoir, 1972, p. 39].

Social policies for the aged in the United States are a failure. This failure is socially constructed and is based on our attitudes toward the aged, as well as our political, economic, and social structures. The dominant view of the aged, which many of the elderly share, is that they are unproductive and dependent persons whose lives are steadily deteriorating. To the extent that this view reflects reality, that reality is determined largely by society. The problem was described poignantly and forcefully by Simone de Beauvoir (1972) when she observed that people enter old age "with empty hands." Society's role in this, she added, is "morally atrocious."

Politics, economics, and social structure have far more to do with the role and the status of the aged than does the aging process and its effects on the individual. Most important are economic policies, particularly those relating to employment and retirement.

221

But also of great importance are the role of special interests in the policy-making process and the extreme fragmentation of policy-making responsibility, which is scattered among federal, state, county, city, regional, and special district jurisdictions and authorities. The price of this fragmentation is high, as McConnell has observed: "The structuring of much of the political system about the array of private associations and other small political units has selected from the values which Americans cherish and has emphasized and given particular effect to narrow and material values. The cost is larger than we normally confess—in limitations on liberty, equality, and . . . public values" (1969, p. 160).

Coupled with this structural diversity is the American ethos that supports a limited role for government, as exemplified by the adage: "That government is best which governs least." More recently, this ethos has been described as the "American reluctance to seek public solutions . . . if there is any possibility of private solutions" (Heidenheimer, Heclo, and Adams, 1975, p. 226). It has been argued that European political structures and culture are more conducive to social change and public planning; certainly they provide less opportunity for special interests to sway policy decisions.

The pluralism that characterizes the American political system, considered by many to be one of its strengths, leads to the belief that the best public policies are those that result from the clash of various special interests; this belief is predicated on the false assumption that the public interest is represented by the congerie of special interests competing for policy control. Pluralism allows interest groups' preferences to replace citizen-based preferences. Interest group pressures and the fragmentation of policy-making responsibilities inhibit broad social change—instead channeling policies in incremental directions. Once a policy is established, organized and resourceful special interests, rather than the largely unrepresented general public, have the advantage in terms of structural power and influence. By contrast, "In less fragmented political systems, policy makers, without disregarding the issues of special interest to particular groups . . . deal from positions of greater strength with the broad policy guidelines which affect everyone in general and no one in particular" (Heidenheimer, Heclo, and Adams, 1975, p. 185). But in the United States, policy inertia is the rule, particularly when it is a question of altering income distribution or tax burdens and benefits. Once a policy is established, change is extremely difficult to effect because "so much is invested in building the consensus [that] the mechanism exhibits little capacity for moving that consensus [and] overcoming the extreme disaggregation in policy" (p. 262).

Historically, state and local governments have been more conservative than the federal government in the initiation of social reforms. States and localities are highly subject to localized interest-group pressure since political choices are made close to home and the cost of such decisions is often immediately experienced through direct taxation. Thus, it has been federal politics and the financial inducement of federal policies that have pulled state and local governments in new directions. Regrettably, new federalism has diluted this source of political vigor and national vision precisely at a time when fiscal crises and taxpayer revolts are creating a demand for cutbacks in social programs at state and local levels. The consequences are likely to be a retreat from policies that included some benefits for the most disadvantaged.

But what has been the overall effect of these social and ideological forces on policies for the aged in the United States? What are the common threads in Social Security, Medicare, Medicaid, food stamps, housing policies, Title XX (social services) and the Older Americans Act? The most important conclusion to be drawn about these policies and the many others designed to benefit the aged directly or indirectly is that they are not meeting the needs of the aged. The policies are largely symbolic and reflect dominant perspectives about the aged. They tend to segregate the aged, often with the poor, as a special class within society. Based on the concept that the aged are in need of services, these policies are often of more benefit to providers of service (physicians, hospitals, banks, mortgage insurance companies) than they are to the aged.

The Older Americans Act reflects many of the problems that characterize other social policies for the aged. This mid-1960s version of national policy for the aged was largely a symbolic gesture that provided limited social and recreational opportunities, "needed" most by middle-income older Americans. The Older

Americans Act reflected the growing visibility of interest groups for the elderly and the awakening of academic, recreational, and social work professionals to a new field of work. The states were originally assigned the major role in determining the needs of the aged and developing plans to meet these needs. The 1973 amendments of the Older Americans Act incorporated a planning and coordination strategy that reflected the growing emphasis on decentralization and local control. Federal revenue sharing and local resources were to provide the needed funds for programs. Thus, as the economic crisis worsened in the 1970s, funding responsibility for services for the aged was shifted from the federal level to the decentralized network of state units and area agencies on aging. By assigning these agencies responsibility to garner local resources in anticipation of continued federal fiscal strain, it was hoped that the growth of federal level economic commitments could be minimized. In the late 1970s, Older Americans Act policies have begun to shift again, abandoning even a limited conception of the social foundations of the problems of the aged and adopting theories that view the problem of old age as one of individual capacity and functioning. In its darkest interpretation, the emerging concern with the functional capacity of the old could preface the time when the aged will be stigmatized even further and forced to be even more dependent on professional certifiers, planners, and providers to obtain needed services—or else will be required to continue working long past current retirement age due to fiscal pressures of the economy. Many assume that Social Security will continue in its present form—a pay-as-you-go system financed by wage earners who may refuse to accept continually escalating Social Security withholding taxes. Such a tax revolt could necessitate the extension of working years well beyond current retirement ages.

The Older Americans Act, like many of the other social policies designed to meet the needs of the aged, receives support and legitimation from theoretical perspectives that have long dominated gerontological research and training in the United States. These perspectives include the disengagement, activity, and developmental theories, all of which contain strong social-psychological components. Another social-psychological theory, lodged within the symbolic interactionist school, is emerging, as are behavioral-exchange, ecological, and environmental theories. However, none of these derives from, or is based upon, macrolevel political economy approaches to old age—approaches that might give theoretical and empirical attention to the social creation of dependency through forced retirement and its functions for the economy (for example, as a contribution to surplus labor), or to the production of senility and the economic, political, and social control functions of such processes. Instead, the individual aspects of aging have been made a primary focus of research, and this emphasis has spawned a research tradition concerned with the social integration of the old, their morale, and adjustment. Underlying many such approaches has been an implicit value bias toward social policies and programs that would enhance the social activity and life satisfaction of the aged, with far less attention being given to the economic, political, and social conditions that largely determine the quality of their lives.

A brief review of these theories of aging and their policy implications will suffice. Disengagement theory prescribes either no policy intervention or interventions that aid the withdrawal of the individual and society from each other. Under such a framework, retirement policies receive legitimation, as do other separatist approaches. Disengagement theory provides the rationalization for a purely symbolic policy because both society and the individual are seen as better off as a consequence of the exclusion of the aged. In contrast, activity theory, which is essentially a (classless and universal) prescription for continued activity in old age, supports policies that assist in the social integration of the aged. Policies focusing on recreational and social activities, that is, life-enhancing rather than life-sustaining activities, are preferred under the tenets of activity theory. In a somewhat similar way, developmental theories, which are based on the "live and let live" principle, emphasize policies that would enable people to maintain their social status throughout the life cycle. This theory calls for highly individualized social policies to meet each individual's needs. Interactionist approaches accord a crucial role to interactional opportunities that build, sustain, or, if necessary, reconstruct the self-esteem of the old, including environmental interventions that foster positive self-images in old age and "aging group consciousness" (Rose and Peterson, 1965). Economic policy is seen as relevant only insofar as it affects socially constructed images of the elderly. None of these approaches, for that matter, begins with the aggregate economic or social condition of the aged; nor does any analyze the economy, legal or political institutions, or the social structure in ways that might lead directly to questions of equity and distributive justice (Estes, 1978). Thus American gerontological perspectives lend little support to social policies that might dramatically alter the distribution of resources in favor of the aged, for such policies are irrelevant to their theories!

Overall, social scientists in the United States have effectively legitimized incrementalist and individualistic approaches, demonstrating Harvey's observation that "social science formulates concepts, categories, relationships, and methods which are not independent of existing social relationships" (Harvey, 1973, p. 125). These social relationships link the social scientist with the social structure (Gouldner, 1970). The most important implication of this is that "the concepts are the product of the very phenomena they are designed to describe" (Harvey, 1973, p. 125).

The conservative role of social science has been a sore point for the Gray Panthers, as illustrated by their public and somewhat bitter criticism of the profession of gerontology: "Gerontology has assumed the deterioration of the aged, and has attempted to describe it in terms which ignore the social and economic factors which in large measure precipitate that deterioration. By reifying the attribute 'old,' gerontology reinforces societal attitudes which view older people as stuck in an inevitable chronological destiny of decay and deterioration. . . . When persons who are old, poor, and stigmatized by society become objects of gerontological research, they are seen as problems to society, rather than as persons experiencing problems created by the society. The natural result of such research is to suggest ways in which older people may adjust to society, rather than how society might be changed to adjust to the needs of older people" (Gray Panthers, 1977). The efforts of the Gray Panthers and other aging-based organizations to confront and redirect societal processing and treatment of the aged are critical to the very necessary construction of a new reality about old age. The central contention of this book, at least, is that aging is something that is done to the chronologically old; that is to say, aging "is not a biological transformation . . . it is a political transformation" (Comfort, 1976b, p. 28).

Additional social aspects of aging posited early in this book were that the experience of old age depends largely upon how others react to the aged; that social context and cultural meanings are crucial influences on this experience; and that older persons individually are powerless to alter their social status and condition because their problems and the appropriate remedies are for the most part defined by the dominant members (the structural interests) of society. Since the labels and definitions applied to any group in society result from reciprocal relationships in which the relative power, class, and social status of interactants play a part, the aged cannot unilaterally alter their relationship to the rest of the society. Nevertheless, the active resistance of the elderly to labels applied to them may contribute to altering the unjust treatment so often accorded them. And as noted by Geiger, current attitudes toward the aged, far from appearing by accident, are "a product of a social structure and a political economy that disposes of people as if there were not enough economically productive work to go around" (1976, p. 5).

Strategies for Failure

What then can we say about the requisite construction of a new reality about old age? It calls for a new perception of old age and a clear understanding of the social, economic, political, and cultural factors that create the very problems now being assiduously discovered by social scientists and policy makers. It calls for a new research agenda as well. Without knowledge about those facets of old age that are socially produced and more knowledge about economic contributions and consequences of aging in the United States, policies for and attitudes toward the aged are likely to continue as symbolic gestures aiding the structural interests that dominate the political scene. It calls for an appreciation which a true "sociology of knowledge" in gerontology might provide in understanding the scholar's and policy maker's contribution to the transformation of objective conditions into public problems and policies (Gusfield, 1976). Further, and even more important, it calls for a true "sociology of knowledge" in gerontology that would make it possible to understand how the scholar and policy maker transform objective conditions into public problems and policies.

America's social policies for the aged are structurally segregated, particularistic policies that tend to separate the old from others in the society. One issue here is whether the "insistence on the special programs just for [older persons creates] tension between [them] and the rest of society" (Etzioni, 1976, p. 29). But the main problem with such an approach is that its rationale has often been predicated upon demeaning images of the aged, and it explicitly invokes negative stereotypes in order to secure resources for the elderly. The deleterious consequences of any process that encourages the portrayal of a social group as impotent, frail, disabled, demented, or dependent cannot be overestimated. As previously noted, the labeling of social groups conditions the way others react tó them. Thus, the negative imagery associated with the aged may not only damage the psychological self-esteem of the aged themselves but severely impair their capacity as a group to engage in interest-group politics and thereby gain their just share of resources.

Other consequences of the separatist ideology are that, by setting the aged apart from the rest of society, it makes them accessible as targets for blame, as well as stigmatization. Age-based approaches that rely on adverse labeling of those sixty years of age and older may increase resentment toward the aged. Society easily comes to look upon the elderly population as an economic and social albatross. Such perceptions exemplify a case of blaming the victim—that is, blaming the aged for economic hardships that are actually a consequence of larger economic and structural factors in the United States and the world economy—among them, involuntary retirement and an economy plagued by inflation and recession. Separatist policies, therefore, have the potential effect of increasing the backlash against the aged.

Conceptions of older persons as unproductive stem from the American belief that only those who work for pay are productive. But older persons are forcibly made "unproductive" by mandatory retirement policies. (It should be noted that all the legislative fanfare about abolishing mandatory retirement has succeeded in delaying this occurrence only from age sixty-five to seventy—and this extension does not apply to all categories of workers.) Such socially created unproductiveness in turn makes the old dependent on society. What is not recognized is that involuntary retirement is a kind of coercive unemployment that aids the economy by reducing unemployment among younger workers. To blame the aged for their forced dependency is to misunderstand the social causation of their condition.

Other examples of "blaming" the aged are found in current controversies over Social Security and health care costs (Samuelson, 1978a). Recent legislation to assure the financial soundness of the Social Security System has resulted in significant increases in the Social Security taxes levied on both employee and employer. What is important about Social Security financing is that it derives solely from taxation related to wage-earning employment. Revenues from corporate taxes, capital gains, dividends, or other benefits of corporate investment are excluded from Social Security taxes. The Congress of the United States, in contrast to a number of other countries, has rejected the principle of supplementing Social Security taxes from general revenues.

As a result, the average wage earner in the United States experiences Social Security as a form of regressive taxation, and the young or middle-aged worker may blame the elderly for the burdens created by its financing mechanism. The fact that inflation and the continuing refusal of Americans to draw on general revenues to stabilize Social Security are major sources of the wage earner's financial hardship is easily overlooked in the face of much simpler explanations. Again, under a separatist ideology it is easier to blame the aged than to try to comprehend the complex and oblique processes by which social expenses are generated.

Such blaming of the aged justifies limiting expenditures and benefits for them to lower-than-subsistence levels. Workers at the same time are encouraged not to believe that an adequate retirement income can be provided through Social Security withholding taxes. Thus, current Social Security financing methods serve as a way of using members of society as agents for controlling the potential expansion of income supports for the aged.

In the same way, discussions of escalating health costs almost invariably lead to accusations that Medicare—and hence, by implication, the elderly population—is the culprit. It is simply ignored that increases in hospital bills and physician fees account for more than 50 percent of the increase in costs over the past fifteen years, and more than 70 percent of the spiraling increases of the last few years. It is also overlooked that third-party payment mechanisms contain built-in incentives to expand the scope and number of services provided (and costs incurred) and that fraud and abuse by providers have cost billions in the Medicare and Medicaid programs (U.S. Senate, 1976b). Older persons have little control over the services they are provided. It is the physician, after all, who orders the tests, prescribes the drugs, orders the hospitalization, and performs the surgery. It is likely that over 70 percent of medical care costs are physician generated. Rather than attributing rising health costs to the demands of the aged, society should place the blame squarely at the door of the incentive structures—reimbursement mechanisms, for example—and a system that makes the provision of health services increasingly profitable to a growing segment of the private economic sector (Ehrenreich and Ehrenreich, 1970).

The crucial dilemma surrounding the politics of old age, however, is whether any disadvantaged group in society can gain access to the resource system without itself becoming a special interest, given the fact that American social policies are determined by bartering among the most vigorous and powerful interest groups. Part of the answer may lie in collective efforts by disadvantaged groups and members of the general population, pressing for universalistic approaches to such shared social problems as poverty (Binstock, 1977; Etzioni, 1976). Examples might be income maintenance policies that would define and, where necessary, provide a given level of income to Americans of all ages and social groups and health security policies that would provide a floor of basic medical coverage regardless of age or other special attributes. Social policies that are not age based would minimize the adverse labeling—often officially legitimated—of those over sixty years of age.

Social policies for the aged in the United States are characterized by policy segmentation and organizational constraint. The potential success of the Older Americans Act and other federal programs for the aged has been jeopardized by the creation of separate departments and government agencies to deal with different facets of the problems of a single population group. The situation in which the Administration on Aging finds itself offers a good example of this problem. As a separate agency within the Department of Health, Education, and Welfare, it operates independently of the Health Care Financing Administration (which administers both the Medicare and Medicaid programs), and it is also distinct from the Social Security Administration, which administers the Old Age and Survivors Insurance Program, along with the Supplementary Security Income program. It is of course separate from the departments of Housing and Urban Development, Transportation, Labor, and Agriculture, all of which administer major programs directly affecting the elderly, as well as from the Veterans Administration, which provides long-term care for many elderly veterans and handles various veteran benefit programs.

In addition, Congress failed to grant sufficient authority to the very organization—the Administration on Aging—that it established to carry out the objectives of the Older Americans Act. Its objectives relate to health, housing, employment, recreation, retirement, community, and social services, which are dealt with by at least a dozen federal departments and independent agencies. It was not until the 1978 reauthorization of the Older Americans Act that language was inserted to require the Administration on Aging to coordinate with these various governmental agencies on the federal level, with the exception of those administering general revenue sharing and Title XX social services. The problem is equally serious in Congress, where dozens of committees and subcommittees deal with the problems of the aged in a piecemeal, fragmented fashion.

This policy segmentation results in an inability to treat any major problem coherently and holistically, and what then occurs is growing public skepticism about the ability of government programs to solve social problems—a skepticism that not only justifies reductions in resource allocations but also gives support to the various solutions that interest groups, providers, and professionals bring forward. In fact, the more complex the problem appears, the more willing the public is to permit discretion to policy makers and experts who claim to have answers—and the more willing the public is to accept the continual failure of those policies because it comes to assume that the problem is so complex as to defy solution anyway. Perhaps most important, policy segmentation causes the public elderly to experience the political world as a series of distinct events and to look upon the environment as basically unpredictable. Not surprisingly, as the public experiences a complex and difficult social problem, such as aging, it becomes increasingly vulnerable to the actions of politicians and interest groups (Douglas, 1971).

Another aspect of policy segmentation is that organizations frequently do not have jurisdiction over areas that are vital to their assigned responsibilities. Welfare agencies, for example, have little authority over the employment resources essential to getting their clients off welfare rolls. Organizational effectiveness is largely determined by organizational jurisdiction. As Edelman has described it: "The names for jurisdictional allocations constitute one of the most potent devices for divorcing organizational accomplishments from their symbolic evocations" (1977, p. 90). The Administration on Aging provides a classic illustration of this problem.

A related problem is that services strategies encourage the breaking down of policy interventions into specialized categorical services to meet individual needs, thereby increasing fragmentation of service provision and preventing an integrated attack on the multifaceted and complex problems of the old person. This specialization itself produces ever-growing classes of service-provider specialists, leads to continual conflicts between public and private agencies, and creates a requirement for adminstrative mechanisms to rationalize and coordinate the many different services and levels of care for which new needs are discovered or manufactured. Again, while the goal of the Older Americans Act was to coordinate services for the aged, the act instead fostered fragmentation of services, and this in two ways—by segregating the aged from younger persons in many, if not most, of the services provided and by establishing separate and, until 1978, uncoordinated titles within the act that frequently have been in competition with one another (for example, between the area planning and nutrition program).

America's social policies for the aged predominantly fall into a services strategy that aids in the maintenance of social harmony and the preservation of existing social-class distinctions. Human services strategies reflect different classes of "deservingness" and entitlements among the aged that in turn correspond to different socioeconomic statuses. Nelson (1978) cites government policies for (1) the "marginal aged" (the "undeserving poor"); (2) the downwardly mobile aged, belonging to the middle and lower-middle classes and newly poor in old age (the "deserving poor"); and (3) the integrated aged, belonging to the middle and upper classes (the nonpoor).

Most services policies tend to favor the downwardly mobile aged, in large part because they are thought of as both deserving and deprived; in addition they have become increasingly organized and are able to press their demands on legislators. The integrated aged have the resources to permit their relatively "unrestricted access to public and private resources" (Nelson, 1978, p. 3) without the necessity of government intervention. The "undeserving" marginal aged are assisted largely through income maintenance policies such as Supplementary Security Income (which does not provide income even at the prevailing poverty level established by the federal government) and health policies that, while highly variable from state to state, consistently encourage removal of the elderly poor from society—first through impoverishment because of inadequate income maintenance policies and then through institutionalization. Medicaid, for example, automatically covers nursing home care, but coverage for home health care is a state option.

The access of the most needy and marginal aged to extant services is restricted by lack of income, transportation, and education, as well as by insufficient knowledge of how to manipulate the system. In contrast, the downwardly mobile elderly, who are more knowledgeable and have more education than the marginal aged, are better able to manage and to take advantage of available benefits. In fact, the services strategy has been designed to meet the needs of the recently deprived aged, since it provides exactly the kinds of services that enable them to maintain their middle-class life-styles. These are "life-enhancing services" that are aimed at enlarging social opportunities (Nelson, 1978, p. 22) rather than life-support services needed by the aged poor. The congregate meals program (which is mainly lauded because of the opportunities it provides for socialization) and senior center programs under the Older Americans Act are examples of life-enhancing services, as are the services that provide access to other needed services under the area planning strategy. Thus, a major consequence of America's services policies is the perpetuation of existing social-class differences; they sustain stratification in that they do not alter the distribution of prestige, income, or other critical resources among or to the aged.

Service strategies are increasingly characterized by the new federalism philosophy that fosters universal eligiblity instead of targeting resources to particular subpopulations of the elderly. Because universal eligibility works to the advantage of those who have the most knowledge about and access to services, it "inherently favors those who . . . are not necessarily in greatest need" (Nelson, 1978, p. 19). Thus, the remedial effects of the already limited services for the most needy are diluted at the outset.

The Older Americans Act reflects this trend toward universal entitlement by granting automatic eligibility at age sixty. Similarly, the 1975 reform of Title XX of the Social Security Act broadened entitlement criteria so that consumers from all classes now have an increasing stake in these services (Gilbert, 1977, p. 624). As Gilbert points out, the percent of Title XX service recipients who are not on welfare has increased significantly relative to those who are on welfare because of the broadened eligibility permitted under Title XX. Given the initial 2.5 (now 2.9) billion dollar national ceiling on Title XX appropriations and the expanded entitlement, the poor must compete for services with other classes of potential recipients. And, "for the aged this means that more nonpoor will compete with, and will receive more services relative to, the poor aged" (Nelson, 1978, p. 24).

The services strategy has serious implications for America's aged because it fosters unequal power relationships between recipients and providers of service. In addition, it creates dependency on two levels: first, for the aged themselves and second, for the society as a whole.

First, the aged who are economically prohibited from creating their own choices and options and who must depend on service providers for minimal assistance quickly learn that they must be cooperative (perhaps even submissive) to receive services. Publicly funded social services are more than systems for distributing services; they are systems of *social relationships* that reflect and bolster power inequities between experts and lay persons, as well as between providers and recipients of service. An increased emphasis on the services solution also means a greater degree of bureaucratization. This is likely to increase the alienation and isolation of the elderly client population, since they must negotiate their way through complex organizations in order to receive services. Further, services that might contribute to the independence of the old (for example, home health care) are given low priority.

Second, policies that provide for the jurisdictional expansion of service providers and middle-level bureaucrats are likely to increase the general public's dependency on services. Thus, social services previously rendered by other institutions (for example, family or church) now come to be performed by paid providers. This leads to further atrophy of traditional support systems, and a vicious circle is thus created that allows the expansionary tendencies of human services professions and industries free rein.

Services strategies in general, and those for the aged in particular, tend to stigmatize their clients as recipients in need, creating the impression that they have somehow failed to assume responsibility for their lives. The needs of older persons are reconceptualized as deficiencies by the professionals charged with treating them, regardless of whether the origins of these needs lie in social conditions over which the individual has little or no control, in the failings of the individual, or in some policy-maker's decision that a need exists.

In addition, services strategies may inadvertently exacerbate the problems for which they are the policy-prescribed solution. The adverse effects that medical treatment can produce (physician-created disease) have long been recognized, and some critics believe that the ill effects of medical care exceed its benefits (Illich, 1977). Similar questions have been raised about the efficacy of social services (Edelman, 1977; McKnight, 1977; Blenker, 1969). Has the growing number of social workers been associated with an in-

crease in family breakups? Why are we spending more and more
on education while our children learn less and less? "The question
is not whether we get less service for more resources. Rather, it
is . . . whether we get the reverse of what the service system is supposed to produce" (McKnight, 1977, p. 112). Yet, the longer the
services conception of the problems and solution persists—and
particularly in a market economy where profits can be made in
human service delivery—the greater the incentives for providers
to expand the net of individual needs for which they can provide
services.

Finally, services approaches are likely to inhibit thinking
about the problems of the aged as related to (or concomitant with)
larger social or economic conditions. This occurs because service
policies individualize problems. And when the needs of an individual are converted into deficiencies requiring the manufacture
and provision of services, his or her problems become isolated
from their social context. McKnight notes the strong effect of this
individualization of the problem "upon [a] citizen's capacities to
deal with cause and effect. If I cannot understand the question or
the answer—the need or the remedy—I exist at the sufferance of
expert systems . . . I am the object rather than the actor. My being
is as a client rather than [as a] citizen" (1977, pp. 110–111).

*Social policies under consideration for the 1980s will continue the
trend toward indirect services.* Government-financed service strategies
for the aged are largely based upon the theory that direct services
are not as necessary as the more indirect services that link and provide access for the client to the (theoretically) already available services. The new emphasis of the 1978 Older Americans Act Amendments on long-term care reinforces the services strategy as the best
policy solution, while also strengthening the notion that aging is
a decremental process that requires interventions focusing on the
biological and not the social aspects of old age. The return to the
biological metaphor as a means of describing the problems of the
elderly (Freeman, 1978) is consonant with the growing national
concern over economic scarcity that has made it increasingly imperative to find intervention strategies that will not add to either
the costs or the expectations of the public. There is also an emerging consensus among policy makers, professionals, and govern-

ment agencies that Older Americans Act agencies should provide an alternative to the institutional-care bias of current federal health policies—Medicare, for example, provides coverage for hospitalization but virtually none for outpatient home health services unless preceded by a hospitalization period, and Medicaid provides much more coverage for hospital and nursing home care than for home health care.

Enlightened as policies for community-based and long-term care may appear, early and growing indications of the Administration on Aging's role in this policy arena do not suggest that the aged themselves will receive many direct benefits. As introduced in the 1978 reauthorization bill, long-term care is being developed as another "indirect" service; the key "services" would be geriatric screening, assessment, and case management. Demonstration programs are being instituted to develop these screening, assessment, and management aspects of long-term care. Often referred to as "personal advocacy," this strategy is likely to foster the development of yet another class of professional troubleshooters who will siphon off a large proportion of the appropriated funds. The costs of such services are likely to be abridged not only by salaries for professionals and paraprofessionals to certify eligibility and manage the aged, but also by the cost of developing yet another set of bureaucracies to house these workers and develop the technology to detect the eligible degree of disability to qualify for services.

Other prospects are that the current long-term care strategy will lead to: (1) the "medicalization" of the problems of the aged, which engenders a perception of their problems as largely physiological, biological, and inevitably decremental; (2) a growing emphasis on individual and case-by-case remedies, an emphasis that will divert attention from the broader economic and social problems of the elderly; (3) a new form of stigmatization of the aged because application of the "vulnerability," "disability," and "frailty" labels in current usage may become a requirement for service eligibility under such a strategy; (4) the increasing isolation of the aged from the rest of society, as their problems come to be processed, screened, and managed through special age-segregated diagnostic agencies; (5) an expansion of the network of social control mechanisms affecting the aged, for the aged who seek assistance may be required to accept such damaging labels as "frail" or "disabled" in order to receive services (Estes and others, 1978)— the threat of which might reduce service demand by entitled age, while also encouraging the dependency of those who receive services; and (6) the potential infringement of the civil liberties of the aged who may be precipitously labeled mentally or physically unfit (possibly without due process) in the rush of program enthusiasm and altruism (Cohen, 1978).

From an economic perspective, the outcomes of indirect service policies will be no more positive. If left in the hands of certifiers and case management officials, these policies will simply produce burgeoning demands for personnel to certify the eligibility of more and more elderly people. Further, there is a serious potential cost boomerang in discovering (or creating by certification) increased numbers of disabled in the population, for this of course could result in more, not less, institutionalization. The bleak truth is that, without a clear federal commitment to direct services that include structural incentives for rehabilitation of the elderly and for supporting their maintenance in their communities, no amount of diagnostic screening or follow-up is likely to help.

The social needs of the aged, then, are defined in ways compatible with the organization of the American economy. The effect of a services strategy is to transform these needs into government-funded and industry-developed commodities for specific economic markets, commodities that are then consumed by the elderly and their "servants." As categories of need are selected for service intervention, these needs are seen as distinct from the system of the production and distribution of wealth that is largely responsible for the needs in the first place. As the focus of attention is shifted from system inequities to individual problems, the blame for the inadequacies of the economic system is displaced onto the aged and the poor (Kincaid, 1973).

Thus a services policy treats the problems of the aged, their illness, and needs independent of their social causes, while positing solutions in the consumption of services. Also, the legitimation of experts to treat only those aspects of the problem to which services are aimed results in a fragmented divisibility of problem-conception and the inadequacy of problem-solving efforts. Such policies serve the multiple functions of obscuring the social and environmental origins of social problems and facilitating the economic growth and expansion of human services technologies, industries, and professions, while isolating problem individuals through categorical and separatist policies that ultimately "pit" disadvantaged groups against one another.

Also disturbing is the trend toward policies (for instance, coordination and functional assessment) that institutionalize indirect services, for their major purpose appears to be the economic functions they provide in the employment of largely white middle-class human service and professional-managerial workers. The "indirectedness" of social services is one key to understanding why there is growing frustration among the aged, the public, and policy-makers; precisely as programs for the aged appear on the ascendancy, there appears to be little tangible result.

But then, services policies are instituted not so much to produce results as to provide a substitute for adequate income maintenance policies. Regrettably, analyses that might expose the conditions of the aged in America remain subordinate to the untested but unshakeable confidence of policy makers that services will solve all problems. Such approaches will probably result in the development of human service monopolies (O'Connor, 1973) that will challenge and eventually control the resources and power structures of the relatively competitive market of small private agencies now supported under the Older Americans Act.

None of these developments will alter the status or condition of the aged. In fact, if the development of "services" continues along current lines, they will remain frustratingly marginal in their capacity to touch the aged. The "services" of planning and coordination (now major emphases of the Older Americans Act) have only indirect effects on the lives and experiences of the aged—and the same will be true of the screening, assessment, and case management services being developed as a consequence of the 1978 amendments to the Older Americans Act. Thus the likelihood is that pressures to expand services will continue to be channeled into "broker" services that effectively augment the resources of providers and the power of professionals (planners, case managers, eligibility certifiers) but that ultimately only place new bureaucratic

barriers between the aged and the government-financed services
that they are supposed to receive.

As the government provides more and more service-related
resources and as the dependency ratio among the elderly increases,
coupled with continuing inflation and recession at all levels of government, politicized demand is likely to escalate service demand—
further expanding the resources, power, and profits of service
agencies and industries and legitimating the professions that provide the indirect social planning, assessment, screening, and case
management services. Thus there will be pressures on the federal
government to develop and expand policies for the aged from the
structural interests that have the most to gain from these policies,
and the continued and very legitimate dissatisfaction of the aged,
whose condition the government policies do not seem to touch. In
light of these demands and the predictable failure of current policies for the aged, several outcomes are possible. A backlash against
the elderly may weaken support for future intervention efforts on
their behalf, given what appears to be their unending demands;
and/or the notion may arise that a crisis exists, that this "crisis" must
be worse than formerly imagined, and that what is needed is more
resources for the same policy strategy. In the latter case the inability of social policies to ameliorate the problems of the aged will
provide the rationale for ever-increasing demands by growth industries of providers and professions that stand to benefit from
servicing the needs of the aged—whether or not they alleviate their
suffering. Thus, the belief that a crisis exists calls forth new solutions, which generate further crises. Crises of this kind do not
necessarily reflect actual demands or needs, but may indicate successful shaping of popular "demand" for symbolic and political
purposes (Edelman, 1977).

A New Vision of Aging

What can be concluded from my examination of the aging
enterprise? Will it be possible to develop effective policies without
a new perception of old age? Will it be possible to radically alter
our vision of aging and the aged in America? I believe that policy
changes are essential on three levels. At the first and most impor-

tant level would be major shifts in perceptions and structural align-
ments, altering both the objective condition of the aged and the
social processes by which policies are made and implemented. At
the second or middle level would be shifts in current major policies
and programs to more effectively meet the needs of the aged—
income maintenance (Social Security, Supplemental Security Income, food stamps), health care (Medicare, Medicaid), and housing
(low-income housing assistance, rent supplements, housing for the
elderly, property tax relief). At the third level would be incremental changes and fine tuning of the eighty or more federal programs
of potential benefit to the aged. My preference is for change on
all three levels, but with primary emphasis on the first.

Policies to facilitate intergenerational bonding and support,
as well as the genuine economic independence and raised social
status of the aged, are imperative, and these would require changes
at the *first level*—namely, an adoption of universalist policies and
principles that would not place the aged in a separate (and potentially unequal) status but would instead eradicate the structural segregation of aging policies from those for other groups in the society. In this sense, my policy recommendations are similar to those
of the Carnegie Council on Children with respect to universal entitlement. After reviewing the constitutional guarantees of freedom of speech, religion, and assembly and the gradual development of such universal entitlements as free public education in the
nineteenth century and unemployment insurance, workers compensation, and Social Security in the twentieth century, the council
observed:

> This concept—sometimes known as universal en-
> titlement—contrasts with another principle of public policy
> which we have repeatedly found unsound—the concept of
> special programs for special people. (One observer has
> called them poor programs for the poor people.) They are
> targeted at specific groups implicitly or explicitly defined
> as inadequate, who deserve help not by right but only
> because of the humanitarian kindness of the donors and
> only as long as the recipients demonstrate their worthiness,
> gratitude, and compliance. These programs—of which wel-
> fare is the classic example—stigmatize their recipients and

commonly subject them to special investigations, tests, requirements, and restrictions. In the short run, special programs for the poor may remain necessary, but the long-range goal of family policy should be to include their recipients in programs that are universal [Keniston and the Carnegie Council on Children, 1977, p. 77].

This book subscribes to the principle of equity that would provide benefits corresponding to relative differences in need (Nelson, 1978), and it also subscribes to Rawls' (1971) conception of social justice, which argues that differences in life prospects are just if the greater expectations of the more advantaged improve the expectations of the least advantaged and that the basic structure of society is just throughout provided that the advantages of the more fortunate further the well-being of the least fortunate. Society's structure is perfectly just provided that the prospects of the least fortunate are as great as they can be.

To achieve equity for the aged it is essential to work jointly on the structural and process levels wherein the social construction of reality emerges. Since current social policies for the aged construct reality in ways that help to maintain existing social-class arrangements, structural changes must begin with income, retirement, and employment policies that at present accentuate class differences among the elderly. Income guarantees are required as a matter of right for every American citizen. Full employment is a national imperative as well, because present levels of unemployment cut the flow of money into Social Security, reduce the income of millions of potential wage earners, and in general contribute to human misery. As a result of forced retirement, the elderly have to rely on publicly financed state benefits and through this reliance are "trapped into poverty" (Walker, 1978, p. 5). Reflecting the "supreme value" that industrial societies place on work, a person's status as independent or dependent is determined largely by his or her participation in the labor market: "The implicit assumption of income maintenance policies [is] that the rewards from work should, in general, be higher than social [that is, governmental] benefits" (p. 9). That work is possible for many, if not most, elderly persons is evident in the continuing activity of physicians, lawyers, farmers, and self-employed businessmen well past the conventional retirement age of sixty-five.

The work ethic in America essentially determines how resources will be apportioned for the elderly, reinforcing class differences forged by a person's lifelong location in the class structure and his or her accompanying employment status. Ignored is the fact that the aged are not at fault for their retirement; in fact, retirement policies aid economic development and have been a requirement of industrialized nations. The aged are not personally at fault for their longevity or for the inflation that has eradicated their savings. Regrettably, as Ackley has pointed out, "There is no recognized constitutional right to the basic necessities of life . . . [and this] failure to recognize a right to subsistence stems directly from a refusal to acknowledge the part played by government in creating the conditions of poverty" (1978, pp. 4, 6).

Employment policies must treat seriously the right of all Americans to work at any age past minority. Similarly, definitions of "deservingness" and productiveness in old age must not be based on the employment status of the elderly. Federal employment policies for the aged have been described as virtually nonexistent (Batten and Kastenbaum, 1976). For example, the few references of the National Commission for Manpower Policy to older workers have usually been to the small employment and volunteer programs for the elderly under the Older Americans Act. As Batten and Kastenbaum show, the de facto federal policy "goes something like this":

> Social Security and Supplementary Security Income are viewed as the major income support sources for most Americans once they retire. Other supports such as Medicare, Medicaid, food stamps, and social services are thought to provide adequately for our older population.
>
> Older workers are presumed to retire at age sixty-five or earlier.
>
> Americans between the ages of forty and sixty-four are presumed to be gainfully employed. Their unemployment rates tend to be low. Whatever vicissitudes they encounter in the labor force are by and large left up to them to cope with.
>
> Employment and training programs are considered to be for youth.
>
> Small categorical programs such as the Senior Aide program provide income supplements for the elderly poor which are regarded as adequate [1976, p. 32].

Current employment and retirement policies must be re-
vised in such a way as to lessen the vulnerability of older workers
to unemployment and to abolish forced retirement—without augmenting the surplus labor market so that wage labor is underpaid
and there is a general reduction in the standard of living of American workers. This shift will require commitment to a full employment economy and an adequate floor on universal income maintenance.

Middle-level policy changes would include restoring to the
Social Security Act those provisions for general-revenue financing
that had been in force between 1944 and 1950; establishing a
"floor" of Social Security benefits at least at the level of the Bureau
of Labor Statistics intermediate budget (which provides a meager
$6,738 per year for an elderly couple); obtaining cash grants in
place of food stamps to provide additional income for food stamp
beneficiaries; elevating Supplementary Security Income payments
above the present federal base, which still does not provide income
at the prevailing poverty level (California Congress of Seniors,
1977); and raising income levels for the determination of the poor
and the near poor so that a realistic appraisal of the extent of poverty in America can be made and social policies based on poverty
indexes will not guarantee impoverishment. For, even with the extremely low poverty level currently utilized, "the proportion of
persons unable to afford a minimum adequate diet has not changed"
over the last ten years; it "remains at about 25 percent of the elderly population" (Binstock, 1977, p. 14).

Middle-level health security measures would require national health insurance for all ages, under provisions that
would provide disincentives rather than incentives for increasing
profits (replacing the current incentive structure with one that
gives special attention to the humane care of Medicare as well as
to the health outcomes of such care). Emphasis should be on
chronic illness, disability, and rehabilitation rather than on acute
care. Because of the present malfunctioning medical care system
with its incentives for overuse and profit, these changes will not be
easy. But certain interim measures would help. For example, costly
deductibles and coinsurance could be eliminated from Medicare
and an adequate prescription drug benefit added. The federali-
zation of Medicaid could make available an adequate scope of ben-

efits to all the poor. Finally, a long-term care policy that emphasizes support for the family and the aged (and that is based in the community and limits institutional care to only that which is essential) could be developed.

A national housing policy to meet the needs of the aged is also clearly needed. Various national organizations have emphasized three general principles as essential in this area: (1) housing needs for older Americans cannot be divorced from the needs of the population as a whole, even though the housing needs of the elderly constitute a special and significant component of a national housing goal; (2) a national program focused on meeting the housing needs of the elderly must be flexible, both in the types of housing that are made available and in the income eligibility requirements; and, (3) the special living environment needs of elderly people (for example, medical and social services) must be taken into consideration to prevent their premature institutionalization, and attention must be given to the qualitative aspects of federal housing programs so that communities rather than housing ghettos are constructed (Crowley in U.S. House, Committee on Banking, Finance, and Urban Affairs, 1978). Adoption of these broad principles and their implementation with adequate appropriations is urgently needed to deal with the very serious housing problems facing the elderly today. Equally important is the need for continued housing subsidies until the aged are able to have a decent income in retirement.

Legal services, transportation, homemaker-chores, home health, and advocacy services are clearly needed. In too many communities even the elderly with adequate income are unable to obtain these needed but sometimes absent services; information about them is often not available to the elderly or the services are not responsive to the needs of the aged.

Who controls the services for the individual is critical to the delivery of social services. Services such as Medicare, although inadequate for all needs, provide the individual with more choice and the possibility of obtaining a more adequate range of services than is usually the case when decisions about service availability and access are made by the provider of service. For example, a small cash grant to an individual for the purchase of social services might produce a more effective result than the allocation of funds directly to social agencies providing homecare or transportation services, one means to restore a partial balance of power in the hands of the elderly. The dilemma in such approaches (and the shortcomings) lies in the assumption that the market will naturally respond—that it will hear the perhaps silent and unorganized "demand" for certain types of services and provide them—and in the potential abandonment of institutional change approaches. But my argument here is that there is little to be expected in the way of institutional changes by simply allocating resources to service providers directly. Institutional changes necessitate major structural changes, such as reorganizing the reward system around health care so that decisions about its availability, quality, and financing are not made based on its being a commodity to be sold at a profit. In the short run, as long as the current structural interests hold (and market decisions, profits, and losses weigh most heavily in the calculus of policy making), the structuring of social service provision in the United States will be basically unchanged. My preference would be for allocating the few remaining choices concerning services to the individual, within limits.

Where does this leave the Older Americans Act? Because it does not deal with the fundamental problems facing the aged, changes in the Older Americans Act belong under the category of *third-level* policy changes. Incremental by definition, they are fine-tuning adjustments of existing policies and processes. In the case of the elderly, third-level changes assume continuation of present decentralization and new federalism policies; they assume that the Older Americans Act, Social Security, Supplementary Security Income, food stamps, housing subsidies, and Medicare/Medicaid will remain the framework for national policy for the aged. With regard to the Older Americans Act, Congress, the Department of Health, Education, and Welfare, and the Administration on Aging must give greater attention to the ambiguities in legislative intent and program implementation. The broad and ill-defined objectives of the Act must be replaced with more specific definitions of objectives, target populations, types and costs of services (direct or indirect), and administrative structures. The lack of clarity, for example, in the roles of the Office of Human Development and the Administration on Aging must be eliminated. Another important change would be the abandonment of strategies that support "indirect services," such as coordination and geriatric screening, at the expense of more direct services—for example, legal and income assistance. Greater incentives are needed to foster cooperation in achieving national goals and to lessen duplication of state and local program goals. Finally, the development of a sound data base for a system of performance monitoring and accountability is also essential. Additional third level policy changes include the need to assure that Social Security and Supplementary Security Income payments do not fall below the poverty level for any recipient. Medicaid benefits must be improved to assure greater equity in access to care for the poor. Medicaid eligibility standards should be federalized in order to cover the medically indigent, as well as those receiving public assistance payments. Federal funds and housing subsidies should be modified to reflect more directly the impact of rising food and housing costs for the elderly.

Although policy and program changes are needed at the second and third levels in the short run, the long-range goal must be policies that provide for an adequate income, a job, decent housing, and health care; that alter the objective condition of the aged; and that change the social processes by which social policies are made and implemented in such a way that the public interests, rather than private special interests, are served. To accomplish these objectives requires the development of a comprehensive national policy on aging that does not segregate the elderly, stigmatize them or place them in a dependent and depersonalized status. To achieve such a national policy will require basic changes in our values, in our attitudes, in our behavior, and in our actions toward the elderly.

The choices are clear. It is time that America became dedicated to the task of transforming old age itself and, in the process, to dismantling the aging enterprise.

References

Abel-Smith, B. *The First Thirty Years.* London: H. M. Stationery Office, 1978.

Ackley, S. "A Right to Subsistence." *Social Policy,* 1978, *8,* 3–15.

Administration on Aging, Office of Human Development, U.S. Department of Health, Education, and Welfare. "Clarification of the Administration on Aging's Policy and Information Issuance System." (AOA–IM–75–58.) Washington, D.C.: U.S. Government Printing Office, 1975.

Administration on Aging, Office of Human Development, U.S. Department of Health, Education, and Welfare. "State and Area Agency on Aging Involvement of a Second Operating Year Services Plan." (AOA–TAM–76–34.) Washington, D.C.: U.S. Government Printing Office, 1976a.

Administration on Aging, Office of Human Development, U.S. Department of Health, Education, and Welfare. "Questions and Answers on the Use of Advisory Bodies in the Title III and VII Programs." (AOA–TAM–76–41.) Washington, D.C.: U.S. Government Printing Office, 1976b.

Administration on Aging, Office of Human Development, U.S. Department of Health, Education, and Welfare. "Evaluation of the First-Year Title XX Experience." (AOA–IM–77–69.) Washington, D.C.: U.S. Government Printing Office, 1977.

Administration on Aging, Office of Human Development, U.S. Department of Health, Education, and Welfare. Annual Report for Fiscal Year 1976. Washington, D.C.: U.S. Government Printing Office, 1978.

Aldrich, H. "Visionaries and Villains: The Politics of Designing Interorganization Relations." *Organization and Administrative Sciences,* 1977, *8* (1), 23–40.

Alford, R., and Friedland, R. "Political Participation and Public Policy." *Annual Review of Sociology,* 1975, *1,* 429–479.

Alford, R. *Health Care Politics.* Chicago: University of Chicago Press, 1976.

Applied Management Sciences. *A Study of State Agencies on Aging: Final Report.* Prepared for Administration on Aging. Silver Spring, Md.: Applied Management Sciences, 1975.

Armour, P. K. "Cycle of Social Reform: Community Mental Health Legislation and Its Implementation in England, Sweden, and the U.S." Unpublished doctoral dissertation, University of California, Berkeley, 1978.

Armour, P. K., Estes, C. L., and Noble, M. L. "Problems in the Design and Implementation of a National Policy on Aging: A Study of Title III of the Older Americans Act." In H. E. Freeman (Ed.), *Policy Studies Review Annual.* Vol. 2. Beverly Hills, Calif.: Sage, 1978.

Atchley, R. C. *Social Forces in Later Life.* Belmont, Calif.: Wadsworth, 1972.

Bach, V. "The New Federalism and Community Development." *Social Policy,* 1977, *7,* 32–38.

Bailey, J. *Social Theory for Social Planning.* London: Routledge & Kegan Paul, 1975.

Ball, R. M. *Social Security Today and Tomorrow.* New York: Columbia University Press, 1978.

Baltes, P. B. "Strategies for Psychological Intervention in Old Age." *Gerontologist,* 1973, *13,* 4–5.

Banfield, E. C. *Political Influence.* New York: Free Press, 1961.

Banfield, E. C. "Revenue Sharing in Theory and Practice." *The Public Interest,* 1971 (23), p. 33.

Batten, M. D., and Kastenbaum, S. "Older People, Work, and Full Employment." *Social Policy,* 1976, *7* (3), 30–33.

Beauvoir, S. de. *The Coming of Age.* London: André Deutsch, 1972.

Bechill, W. *Developments and Trends in State Programs and Services for the Elderly: A Survey of Activities at the State Governmental Level in the Field of Aging, 1972–1973.* College Park, Md.: University of Maryland and Senate Special Committee on Aging, 1974.

Becker, H. *The Outsiders.* New York: Free Press, 1963.

Beer, S. H. "The Adoption of General Revenue Sharing: A Case Study in Public Sector Politics." *Public Policy,* 1976, *24,* 127–195.

Beer, S. H. "Federalism, Nationalism, and Democracy in America." *American Political Science Review,* 1978, *72* (1), 9–21.

Benedict R. *Meeting the Needs of the Chronically Impaired Older Persons: A Background and Concept Paper for the Reauthorization of the Older Americans Act.* Washington, D.C.: Administration on Aging, 1978.

"The Beneficent Monster." *Time,* 1978, *111* (24), 24–32.

Bengston, V. L., and Cutler, N. E. "Generations and Intergenerational Relations: Perspectives on Age Groups and Social Change." In R. H. Binstock and E. Shanas (Eds.), *Handbook of Aging and the Social Sciences.* New York: D. Van Nostrand, 1976.

Benton, B., Feild, T., and Millar, R. *State and Area Agency on Aging Intervention in Title XX.* Washington, D.C.: Urban Institute, 1977.

Benton, B., and others. *The Effect of Title XX on Women and Minorities.* Washington, D.C.: Urban Institute, 1977.

Berger, P., and Luckmann, T. *The Social Construction of Reality.* New York: Doubleday, 1966.

Berger, P., and Neuhaus, R. *To Empower People.* Washington, D.C.: American Enterprise Institute, 1977.

Beyer, G. "Revenue Sharing and the New Federalism." *Society,* 1974, *11* (2), 58–61.

Binstock, R. H. *Planning.* Report for the White House Conference on Aging. Washington, D.C.: U.S. Government Printing Office, 1971.

Binstock, R. H. "Interest-Group Liberalism and the Politics of Aging." *Gerontologist,* 1972a, *12,* 265–280.

Binstock, R. H. "The Roles and Functions of State Planning Systems: Preliminary Report on a Nationwide Survey of State Units on Aging." Preliminary report for Administration on Aging. Waltham, Mass.: Florence Heller School for Advanced Studies in Social Welfare, Brandeis University, 1972b.

Binstock, R. H. "Aging and Public Policy: Contemporary Trends and Issues." In J. A. Gaida (Ed.), *Gerontology at Saint Michael's: 1977.* Winooski, Vt.: Saint Michael's College Press, 1977.

Binstock, R. H. "Federal Policy Toward the Aging: Its Inadequacies and Its Politics." National Journal, 1978, *10,* 1838–1845.

Binstock, R. H., and Levin, M. A. "The Political Dilemmas of Intervention Policies." In R. H. Binstock and E. Shanas (Eds.), *Handbook of Aging and the Social Sciences.* New York: D. Van Nostrand, 1976.

Blenker, M. "Service and Survival." *Proceedings of the International Congress of Gerontology,* 1969, *1,* 417–420.

Blumer, H. *Symbolic Interactionism: Perspective and Method.* Englewood Cliffs, N. J.: Prentice-Hall, 1969.

Blumer, H. "Social Problems as Collective Behavior." *Social Problems,* 1971, *18* (3), 298–306.

Borzilleri, T. C. "The Need for a Separate Consumer Price Index for Older Persons: A Review and New Evidence." *Gerontologist,* 1978, *18* (3), 230–236.

Brinnon, S. "Questioning Needs Assessment." Memorandum. Washington, D.C.: U.S. Department of Health, Education, and Welfare, 1975.

Broder, D. *The Party's Over: The Failure of Politics in America.* New York: Harper & Row, 1972.

Brotman, H. B. "The Aging of America: A Demographic Profile." *National Journal,* 1978, *10,* 1622–1627.

Busse, E. W., and Pfeiffer, E. *Behavior and Adaptation in Late Life.* (2nd ed.) Boston: Little, Brown, 1977.

Butler, L., Newacheck, P., and Piontkowski, D. *Dollars and Disability: A Policy Analysis of Low Income and Health.* San Francisco: Health Policy Program, School of Medicine, University of California, 1978.

Butler, R. N. *Why Survive? Being Old in America.* New York: Harper & Row, 1975.

Califano, J. A. "The Aging of America: Questions for the Four-Generation Society." Paper presented at the annual meeting of the American Academy of Political and Social Science, Philadelphia, April, 1978.

"Califano Proposes Progressive Policies for Nation's Elderly." *Aging,* 1978 (385–386), pp. 1–4.

California Congress of Seniors. Resolution. San Francisco: California Association of Older Americans, 1977.

Carp, F. M. "Person-Situation Congruence in Engagement." *Gerontologist,* 1968, *8,* 184–188.

Clark, R. B., Kreps, J., and Spangler, J. "Economics of Aging." *Journal of Economic Literature,* 1978, *16,* 919–962.

Cohen, E. S. "Comment on 'Aging in America: Toward the Year 2000.' " *Gerontologist,* 1976, *16,* 270–275.

Cohen, E. S. "Civil Liberties and the Frail Elderly." *Transaction Society,* 1978, *15* (5), 34–42.

Colfax, J. D., and Roach, J. L. (Eds.). *Radical Sociology.* New York: Basic Books, 1971.

Comfort, A. "Age Prejudice in America." *Social Policy,* 1976a, 7 (3), 3–8.

Comfort, A. *A Good Age.* New York: Crown, 1976b.

Congressional Record. Proceedings and Debates of the 95th Congress, 2nd Session, July 24, 1978, *124* (112).

Connolly, W. E. *The Bias of Pluralism.* New York: Atherton, 1969.

Coser, L. "The Sociology of Poverty." *Social Problems,* 1963, *13,* 140–148.

Cumming, E. "Further Thoughts on the Theory of Disengagement." United Nations Educational, Scientific, and Cultural Organization, *International Social Science Journal,* 1974, *15,* 377–393.

Cumming, E., and Henry, W. E. *Growing Old: The Process of Disengagement.* New York: Basic Books, 1961.

Cutler, N. E. "Resources for Senior Advocacy: Political Behavior and Partisan Flexibility." In P. A. Kerschner (Ed.), *Advocacy and Age.* Los Angeles: University of Southern California Press, 1976.

Dahl, R. *A Preface to the Democratic Theory.* Chicago: University of Chicago Press, 1956.

Douglas, J. *American Social Order.* New York: Free Press, 1971.

Edelman, M. *The Symbolic Uses of Politics.* Urbana: University of Illinois Press, 1964.

Edelman, M. *Politics as Symbolic Action.* Chicago: Markham, 1971.

Edelman, M. *Political Language: Words That Succeed and Policies That Fail.* New York: Academic Press, 1977.

Ehrenreich, B., and Ehrenreich, J. *The American Health Empire.* New York: Random House, 1970.

Ehrenreich, B., and Ehrenreich, J. "Health Care and Social Control." *Social Policy,* 1974, *5* (2), 26–40.

Equal Opportunity Act of 1964, as Amended in 1965. (Public Law 89–253, as Amended.) Washington, D.C.: Office of Economic

Opportunity, U.S. Department of Health, Education, and Welfare, 1965.

Estes, C. L. "Community Planning for the Elderly from an Organizational, Political, and Interactionist Perspective." Unpublished doctoral dissertation, University of California, San Diego, 1972.

Estes, C. L. "Barriers to Effective Community Planning for the Elderly." *Gerontologist,* 1973, *13* (2), 178–183.

Estes, C. L. *Organizational Structures, Goals, Interorganizational Relations, and Innovation: A Selected Review and Analysis.* Monograph submitted to Brandeis University and Administration on Aging, 1974a.

Estes, C. L. "Community Planning for the Elderly: A Study of Goal Displacement." *Journal of Gerontology,* 1974b, *29,* 684–691.

Estes, C. L. "New Federalism and Aging." In U.S. Senate, Special Committee on Aging, *Developments in Aging: 1974 and January-April, 1975.* Report No. 94–998, Part I. Washington, D.C.: U.S. Government Printing Office, 1975a.

Estes, C. L. "Organizational and Political Barriers to Self-Determination by the Elderly in Programs Meant To Serve Them." Paper presented at the annual meeting of the Gerontological Society, Louisville, Ky., October 1975b.

Estes, C. L. "Goal Displacement in Community Planning for the Elderly: Implications for National Policy." In P. Lawton, R. Newcomer, and T. Byerts (Eds.), *Community Planning for an Aging Society.* Stroundsburg, Pa.: Dowden, Hutchinson, and Ross, 1976a.

Estes, C. L. "The Politics of Community Planning for the Elderly." *Policy and Politics,* 1976b, *4,* 51–70.

Estes, C. L. "Revenue Sharing: Implications in Policy and in Aging." *Gerontologist,* 1976c, *16* (2), 141–147.

Estes, C. L. "Political Gerontology." *Transaction Society,* 1978, *15* (5), 43–49.

Estes, C. L., Armour, P. K., and Noble, M. L. "Intent Vs. Implementation: Toward an Analytic Framework for Understanding the Older Americans Act." Paper presented at the annual meeting of the Gerontological Society, San Francisco, October 1977.

Estes, C. L., and Freeman, H. E. "Strategies of Design and Research for Intervention." In R. H. Binstock and E. Shanas (Eds.), *Handbook of Aging and the Social Sciences.* New York: D. Van Nostrand, 1976.

Estes, C. L., and Gerard, L. "Legislative History and Development of the Older Americans Act." Unpublished paper, Department of Social and Behavioral Sciences, School of Nursing, University of California, San Francisco, 1978a.

Estes, C. L., and Gerard, L. "Politics and Policy for the Aged: An Analysis of the 1978 Reauthorization of the Older Americans Act." Unpublished paper, Department of Social and Behavioral Sciences, School of Nursing, University of California, San Francisco, 1978b.

Estes, C. L., and Noble, M. L. *Paperwork and the Older Americans Act: Problems of Implementing Accountability.* Staff information paper prepared for use by the Special Committee on Aging, U.S. Senate. Washington, D.C.: U.S. Government Printing Office, 1978.

Estes, C. L., Shaw, M., and Stunkel, E. *Developments and Trends in Aging: A Survey of Programs, Legislation, and Information Systems in a Sample of States.* Sacramento: California Commission on Aging, 1975.

Estes, C. L., and others. "State and Local Trends in Health Services for the Aging." Paper presented at the National Symposium on Aging, San Francisco, February 1978.

Etzioni, A. "Old People and Public Policy." *Social Policy,* 1976, *7,* 21–29.

Executive Office of the President, Office of Management and Budget. *1978 Catalog of Federal Domestic Assistance.* Washington, D.C.: U.S. Government Printing Office, 1978.

Federal Council on the Aging. *Annual Report: 1977.* Washington, D.C.: Federal Council on the Aging, 1978.

Federal Register. Federal Regulations for Title III of the Older Americans Act, October 11, 1973, *37* (196), 28047.

Feild, T., Millar, R., and Benton, B. *The Effects of Title XX Implementation on the Allocation of Social Services.* Washington, D.C.: Urban Institute, 1978.

Fleisher, D., and Kaplan, B. H. "Factors Associated with Encouraging Older Service Users To Assume Roles as Active Policy Makers." Paper presented at the International Congress of Gerontology, Tokyo, August 1978.

Foltz, A. M. *Uncertainties of Federal Child Health Policies: Impact in Two States.* Hyattsville, Md.: National Center for Health Services Research, U.S. Department of Health, Education, and Welfare, 1978.

Freeman, M. "Limits of the Biological Metaphor." Unpublished paper, Department of Sociology, University of California, Davis, 1978.

Friedland, R., Alford, R. R., and Piven, F. F. "The Political Management of the Urban Fiscal Crisis." Paper presented at the annual meeting of the American Sociological Association, Chicago, September 1977.

Galbraith, J. K. *American Capitalism: The Concept of Countervailing Power.* Boston: Houghton Mifflin, 1952.

Gardner, J. *No Easy Victories.* New York: Harper & Row, 1968.

Gartner, A. "Consumers in the Service Society." *Social Policy,* 1977, *7,* 2–8.

Geiger, H. S. "Some Comfort for Old Age: A Good Age and Prolongevity." *New York Times Book Review,* November 28, 1976, pp. 5–6.

Gerth, H. H., and Mills, C. W. (Trans. and Eds.). *From Max Weber: Essays in Sociology.* New York: Oxford University Press, 1946.

Gilbert, N. "The Transformation of Social Services." *Social Service Review,* 1977, *51,* 624–641.

Gilbert, N., and Specht, H. "Title XX Planning by Area Agencies on Aging: Efforts, Outcomes, and Policy Implications." Working Paper No. 101. Berkeley, Calif.: Institute for Scientific Analysis, 1977.

Gordon, A., and others. "Beyond Need: Toward a Service Society." Unpublished paper, Department of Sociology, Northwestern University, 1974.

Gouldner, A. *The Coming Crisis of Western Sociology.* New York: Basic Books, 1970.

Gray Panthers. Pamphlet distributed at the annual meeting of the Gerontological Society, San Francisco, November 1977.

Gubrium, J. F. (Ed.). *The Myth of the Golden Years.* Springfield, Ill.: Thomas, 1973.

Gusfield, J. "Literary Rhetoric of Science." *American Sociological Review,* 1976, *41,* 1–33.

Hage, J., and Aiken, M. "Program Change and Organizational

Properties: A Comparative Analysis." *Journal of Sociology,* 1967, *73,* 503–519.

Hall, P. M. "A Symbolic Interactionist Analysis of Politics." In A. Effrat (Ed.), *Perspectives in Political Sociology.* Indianapolis: Bobbs-Merrill, 1973.

Harvey, D. *Social Justice and the City.* Baltimore: Johns Hopkins University Press, 1973.

Havighurst, R. J. "Successful Aging." In R. Williams, C. Tibbitts, and W. Donahue (Eds.), *Processes of Aging.* New York: Atherton, 1963.

Heidenheimer, A. J., Heclo, H., and Adams, C. T. *Comparative Public Policy.* New York: St. Martin's, 1975.

Henry, W. "The Theory of Intrinsic Disengagement." In P. F. Hansen (Ed.), *Age with a Future.* Philadelphia: Davis, 1964.

Hochschild, A. R. "Disengagement Theory: Critique and Proposal." *American Sociological Review,* 1975, *40,* 553–569.

Hochschild, A. R. "Disengagement Theory: A Logical, Empirical, and Phenomenological Critique." In J. F. Guberman (Ed.), *Time Roles and Self in Old Age.* New York: Human Sciences Press, 1976.

Honolulu Advertiser, August 25, 1978.

Howenstine, R. A., Miller, J., and Tucker, R. C. *Research on Social Systems and Interagency Relations: A Study of the Area Agencies on Aging.* New Haven, Conn.: Yale University Press, 1975.

Hudson, R. B. "A Political Perspective on Title XX." Unpublished paper, Brandeis University, 1977. (In *Political Perspectives on the Social Services,* forthcoming.)

Human Resources Corporation. *Advocacy in the Field of Aging.* Unpublished report prepared for Administration on Aging. San Francisco: Human Resources Corporation, 1975.

Human Resources Corporation. "Policy Issues Concerning the Minority Elderly." Final Report/Executive Summary submitted to Federal Council on the Aging. San Francisco: Human Resources Corporation, 1978.

Iglehart, J. K. "The Cost of Keeping the Elderly Well." *National Journal,* 1978, *10,* 1728–1731.

Illich, I. *The Medical Nemesis.* New York: Random House, 1977.

Jacob, P. "Autonomy and Political Responsibility." *Urban Affairs Quarterly,* 1975, *2,* 36–57.

Johnson, M. Testimony before the U.S. House of Representatives, Select Committee on Aging. Cincinnati, Ohio, August 1978.

Juster, F. T. (Ed.). *The Economic and Political Impact of General Revenue Sharing.* Washington, D.C.: National Science Foundation, 1976.

Kane, R. L., and Kane, R. A. "Care of the Aged: Old Problems in Need of New Solutions." *Science,* 1978, *200,* 913–919.

Kaplan, M. "The Model Cities Program." Unpublished report prepared for Model Cities. Washington, D.C.: U.S. Department of Housing and Urban Development, 1970.

Keniston, K., and the Carnegie Council on Children. *All Our Children.* New York: Harcourt Brace Jovanovich, 1977.

Kincaid, J. C. *Poverty and Equality in Britain.* Middlesex, England: Penguin Books, 1973.

Kirschner and Associates. *Objective Setting and Monitoring.* Prepared for U.S. Department of Health, Education, and Welfare. Washington, D.C.: U.S. Government Printing Office, 1975.

Lauffer, A. "Area Planning for the Aging." Unpublished draft prepared for Administration on Aging, Washington, D.C., 1974.

Levitan, S. *The Great Society's Poor Law.* Baltimore: Johns Hopkins University Press, 1969.

Lichtman, R. "Symbolic Interactionism and Social Reality: Some Marxist Queries." *Berkeley Journal of Sociology,* 1970, *15,* 75–94.

Livers, P. J. Letter from Director, Bureau of Supplemental Security Income, Social Security Administration, November 2, 1978.

Lovell, C. H., Korey, J., and Weber, C. "The Effects of General Revenue Sharing on Ninety-Seven Cities in Southern California." Unpublished paper, Graduate School of Administration, University of California, Riverside, 1975.

Lowenthal, M. F. "Psychosocial Variations Across the Adult Life Course: Frontiers for Research and Policy." *Gerontologist,* 1975, *15* (1), 6–12.

Lowi, T. *The End of Liberalism.* New York: Norton, 1969.

Lowi, T. *The Politics of Disorder.* New York: Basic Books, 1971.

Lukes, S. *Essays in Social Theory.* New York: Columbia University Press, 1977.

Lyman, S. M., and Scott, M. B. *A Sociology of the Absurd.* New York: Appleton-Century-Crofts, 1970.

McConnell, G. "The Public Values of Private Association." In

R. Pennock and J. W. Chapman (Eds.), *Voluntary Associations.*
New York: Atherton, 1969.

MacIver, Robert N. *The Web of Government.* New York: Macmillan,
1947.

McKnight, J. "Professional Service Business." *Social Policy,* 1977,
8 (3), 110–116.

Maddox, G. L. "Sociological Perspectives in Gerontology Research." In D. Kent, R. Kastenbaum, and S. Sherwood (Eds.),
Research, Planning, and Action for the Elderly. New York: Behavioral Publications, 1972.

Marmor, T. R., and Kutza, E. A. *Analysis of Federal Regulations Related to Aging: Legislative Barriers to Coordination Under Title III.*
Chicago: University of Chicago, 1975.

Marris, P., and Rein, M. *Dilemmas of Social Reform.* Chicago: Aldine,
1967.

Marshall, V., and Tindale, J. A. "Toward a Radical Social Gerontology." Paper presented at the annual meeting of the Gerontological Society, Louisville, Ky., October 1975.

Marx, K. *Das Kapital.* F. Engels (Ed.). Chicago: Regnery, 1961.
(Originally published 1867.)

Matza, D. *Becoming Deviant.* Englewood Cliffs, N.J.: Prentice-Hall,
1969.

Mead, G. H. *Mind, Self, and Society.* Chicago: University of Chicago
Press, 1934.

Mendelson, M. A. *Tender Loving Greed.* New York: Random House,
1975.

Miller, S. M. "The Political Economy of Social Problems: From the
60s to the 70s." Paper presented at the annual meeting of the
Society for Study of Social Problems, New York, August 1976.

Mills, C. W. *The Power Elite.* New York: Oxford University Press,
1956.

Mogulof, M. B. *Citizen Participation: The Local Perspective.* Washington, D.C.: Urban Institute, 1970.

Mogulof, M. B. "Special Revenue Sharing and the Social Services."
Social Work, 1973, *18,* 9–15.

Moon, M. *The Measurement of Economic Welfare: Its Application to the
Poor.* New York: Academic Press, 1977.

Mueller, C. *The Politics of Communication.* New York: Oxford University Press, 1973.

Nathan, R. P., Manvel, A. D., and Calkins, S. E. *Monitoring Revenue Sharing.* Washington, D.C.: Brookings Institution, 1975.

Nathan, R. P., Adams, C. F., and Associates. *Revenue Sharing: The Second Round.* Washington, D.C.: Brookings Institution, 1977.

National Academy of Sciences. *Health Care for American Veterans: Report of the Committee on Health Care Resources in the Veterans Administration.* Washington, D.C.: Assembly of Life Sciences, National Research Council, National Academy of Sciences, 1977.

National Council on the Aging, Inc. *The Myths and Reality of Aging in America.* Washington, D.C.: Louis Harris and Associates, 1975.

National Council on the Aging, Inc. *Title XX of the Social Security Act: A Resource Serving the Needs of Older People.* Washington, D.C.: National Council on the Aging, Inc., 1976.

National Science Foundation. *General Revenue Sharing.* Vol. 4: *Synthesis of Impact and Process Research.* Washington, D.C.: U.S. Government Printing Office, 1975.

Nelson, G. "Perspectives on Social Need and Social Services to the Aged." Unpublished paper, School of Social Welfare, University of California, Berkeley, 1978.

Neugarten, B. L., Havighurst, R. J., and Tobin, S. S. "Personality and Patterns of Aging." *Gaewin,* 1963, *13,* 249–256.

Neugarten, B. L., and others (Eds.). *Personality in Middle and Late Life.* New York: Atherton, 1964.

O'Brien, J., and Wetle, T. T. *Final Report: Analysis of Conflict in Coordination of Aging Services.* Prepared for Administration on Aging. Portland, Ore.: Institute on Aging, Portland State University, 1975.

O'Connor, J. *The Fiscal Crisis of the State.* New York: St. Martin's, 1973.

O'Shea, R. M., and Gray, S. B. "Income and Community Participation." *Welfare in Review,* 1966, *4* (4), 10–13.

Okun, A. M. "Inflation: The Problems and Prospects Before Us." In A. M. Okun, M. Fowler, and M. Gilbert (Eds.), *Inflation: The Problems It Creates and the Policies It Requires.* New York: University Press, 1970.

Older Americans Act of 1965, as Amended. (Public Law 89–73, as Amended.) Washington, D.C.: Administration on Aging, U.S. Department of Health, Education, and Welfare, 1976.

Older Americans Act of 1965, as Amended: Comprehensive Older

Americans Act Amendments of 1978. (Public Law 95–478, as Amended.) U.S. House of Representatives, Conference Report No. 95–1618. Washington, D.C.: U.S. Government Printing Office, 1978.

Perlman, J. "Grass Rooting the System." *Social Policy*, 1976, 7, 4–20.

Perrow, C. "Goals and Power Structures." In E. Freidson (Ed.), *The Hospital in Modern Society*. New York: Free Press, 1963.

Pratt, H. "Symbolic Politics and White House Conference on Aging." *Transaction Society*, 1978, *15* (5), 67–72.

Pressman, J., and Wildavsky, A. *Implementation*. Berkeley: University of California Press, 1973.

Rawls, J. *The Theory of Justice*. Cambridge, Mass.: Harvard University Press, 1971.

Renaud, M. "On the Structural Constraints of State Intervention in Health." *International Journal of Health Services*, 1975, *5* (4), 559–571.

Roemer, R., Kramer, C., and Frink, J. E. *Planning Urban Health Services from Jungle to System*. New York: Springer, 1975.

Roman, P., and Taietz, P. "Organizational Structure and Disengagement: The Emeritus Professor." *Gerontologist*, 1967, 7, 147–152.

Rondinelli, D. A. "Revenue Sharing and American Cities: Analysis of the Federal Experiment in Local Assistance." *Journal of the American Institute of Planners*, 1975, *41* (5), 319–333.

Rose, A. M., and Peterson, W. A. (Eds.). *Older People and Their Social World*. Philadelphia: Davis, 1965.

Rose, L. S., Zorn, F. E., and Radin, B. "Title XX and Public Participation: An Initial Assessment." *Public Welfare*, 1976, *35* (1), 24–31.

Rose, S. M. "Ideology and Urban Planning: The Muddle of Model Cities." Paper presented at the annual meeting of the American Sociological Association, August/September, 1971.

Samuelson, R. J. "Busting the U.S. Budget: The Costs of an Aging America." *National Journal*, 1978a, *10* (7), 256–260.

Samuelson, R. J. "The Elderly: Who Will Support Them?" *National Journal*, 1978b, *10* (43), 1712–1717.

San Francisco Chronicle, October 25, 1978a, p. 9.

San Francisco Chronicle, October 28, 1978b, p. 1.

San Francisco Chronicle, November 30, 1978c, p. 56.

Schooler, K. K., and Estes, C. L. "Differences Between Current Gerontological Theories: Implications for Research Methodology." In D. Kent, R. Kastenbaum, and S. Sherwood (Eds.), *Research, Planning, and Action for the Elderly.* New York: Behavioral Publications, 1972.

Schulz, J. H. *The Economics of Aging.* Belmont, Calif.: Wadsworth, 1976.

Schultz, C. L. "The Role of Incentives, Penalties, and Rewards in Attaining Effective Policy." In R. H. Haveman and H. Margolis (Eds.), *Public Expenditures and Policy Analysis.* Chicago: Markham, 1971.

Scott, R. *The Making of Blind Men.* New York: Russell Sage Foundation, 1970.

Selznick, P. *TVA and the Grass Roots.* Berkeley: University of California Press, 1949.

Silver, G. A. "Politics and Social Policy: Child Health." Report of the Yale Health Policy Project. New Haven, Conn.: School of Medicine, Yale University, 1976.

Silverman, E. B. "New York City Revenues: The Federal and State Role." In R. R. Alcaly and D. Mermelstein (Eds.), *The Fiscal Crisis of American Cities.* New York: Vintage Books, 1967.

Singer, J. W. "A Brighter Future for Older Workers." *National Journal,* 1978, *10,* 1722–1725.

Sjoberg, G., Brymer, R. A., and Farris, B. "Bureaucracy and the Lower Class." *Sociology and Social Research,* 1966, *50,* 325–337.

"Social Services '75 . . . A Citizen's Handbook: Program Options and Public Participation under Title XX of the Social Security Act." Pamphlet. Washington, D.C.: U.S. Government Printing Office, 1975.

Stanfield, R. L. "Services for the Elderly: A Catch-22." *National Journal,* 1978, *10,* 1718–1721.

State and Local Fiscal Assistance Act of 1972: State and Local Fiscal Amendments of 1976. (Public Law 94–488, as Amended.) Washington, D.C.: U.S. Government Printing Office, 1976.

Steinberg, R. M. "Follow the Rules to Red Tape or Blue Ribbons: A Study of Task Deflection and Positive Reinforcement in Delivery of Services to the Elderly by Funding Regulations and Accountability Procedures." Paper presented at the annual meeting of the Gerontological Society, Louisville, Ky., October 1975. Report No. 2 of *A Study of Funding Regulations, Program Agreements, and Monitoring Procedures Affecting the Implementation of Title III of the Older Americans Act.* Los Angeles: Social Policy Laboratory, Ethel Percy Andrus Gerontology Center, University of Southern California, 1975.

Steinberg, R. M. "A Longitudinal Analysis of 97 Area Agencies on Aging." Report No. 3 of *A Study of Funding Regulations, Program Agreements, and Monitoring Procedures Affecting the Implementation of Title III of the Older Americans Act.* Los Angeles: Social Policy Laboratory, Ethel Percy Andrus Gerontology Center, University of Southern California, 1976.

Suchman, E. *Evaluation Research.* New York: Russell Sage Foundation, 1967.

"The Swarming Lobbyists." *Time,* August 7, 1978, *112* (6), 14–22.

Tallmer, M., and Kutner, B. "Disengagement and the Stresses of Aging." *Journal of Gerontology,* 1969, *24,* 70–75.

Thernstrom, S. *Poverty, Planning, and Politics in the New Boston.* New York: Basic Books, 1969.

Thomas, W. I. *The Unadjusted Girl.* Santa Fe, N.M.: Gannor, 1970.

Tobin, S. S., Davidson, S. M., and Sack, A. *Effective Social Services for Older Americans.* Prepared for Administration on Aging. Ann Arbor: Institute of Gerontology, University of Michigan and Wayne State University, 1976.

Tokarz, J. T. "Title XX Social Services: Many Changes, Many Problems." *Grantsmanship Center News,* 1977, *20,* 38–44.

Trela, J. E. "Some Political Consequences of Senior Center and Other Old Age Group Memberships." *Gerontologist,* 1971, *2,* 118–123.

Twaddle, A. C., and Hessler, R. M. *Sociology of Health.* St. Louis: Mosby, 1977.

U.S. Commission on Civil Rights. *The Age Discrimination Study.* Washington, D.C.: U.S. Commission on Civil Rights, 1977.

U.S. Congress, Congressional Budget Office. *Long-Term Care for the Elderly and Disabled.* Washington, D.C.: U.S. Government Printing Office, 1977.

U.S. Congress, Congressional Budget Office. *Share of Federal Expenditures for the Elderly.* Washington, D.C.: U.S. Government Printing Office, 1978.

U.S. Congress, Joint Committee on Internal Revenue Taxation. *General Explanation of the State and Local Fiscal Assistance Act and the Federal-State Tax Collection Act of 1972.* (Public Law 92–512.) U.S. House of Representatives, February 12, 1973.

U.S. Department of Health, Education, and Welfare. *Health United States, 1976–1977.* Washington, D.C.: U.S. Government Printing Office, 1977.

U.S. Department of Health, Education, and Welfare, Social Security Administration. *Social Security Bulletin,* January 1978. Washington, D.C.: U.S. Government Printing Office, 1978.

U.S. Department of Housing and Urban Development. *HUD News,* September 20, 1978, HUD-No. 78–306.

U.S. Department of the Treasury, Office of Revenue Sharing. *General Revenue Sharing—Statistical Summary (1/1/72–6/30/74).* Washington, D.C.: U.S. Government Printing Office, 1975.

U.S. Department of the Treasury, Office of Revenue Sharing. *5th Annual Report of Office of Revenue Sharing.* Washington, D.C.: U.S. Government Printing Office, 1978.

U.S. General Accounting Office. Letter from the Deputy Comptroller General of the U.S. to Congressman Claude Pepper, undated in 1973.

U.S. General Accounting Office. "Local Area Agencies Help the Aging but Problems Need Correcting." Report of the Comptroller General of the U.S. to Administration on Aging, U.S. Department of Health, Education, and Welfare, August 2, 1977. Washington, D.C.: U.S. Government Printing Office, 1977a.

U.S. General Accounting Office. "Home Health—The Need for a National Policy To Better Provide for the Elderly." Report of the Comptroller General of the U.S. to the Congress, December 30, 1977b.

U.S. General Accounting Office. "The 1975 Amendments to the Older Americans Act—Little Effect on Spending for Priority Services." Report of the Comptroller General of the U.S. to the Congress, March 1978.

U.S. House of Representatives, Committee on Appropriations, Subcommittee on the Departments of Labor and Health, Education, and Welfare. Hearings for Fiscal Year 1978. Washington, D.C.: U.S. Government Printing Office, 1977.

U.S. House of Representatives, Committee on Banking, Finance, and Urban Affairs, Subcommittee on Housing and Community Development. Hearings, March 23, 1978.

U.S. House of Representatives, Committee on Education and Labor, Subcommittee on Select Education. Hearings: "Administration on Aging," Washington, D.C., September 17–19, 1963.

U.S. House of Representatives, Committee on Education and Labor, Subcommittee on Select Education. Hearings to Amend the Older Americans Act of 1965, February 8, 1973. Washington, D.C.: U.S. Government Printing Office, 1973.

U.S. House of Representatives, Committee on Education and Labor, Subcommittee on Select Education. Hearings: "Public Law 93–29, Older Americans Comprehensive Services Amendments of 1973 and Related Programs," Washington, D.C., January 30, February 3–4, 1975.

U.S. House of Representatives, Committee on Education and Labor, Subcommittee on Select Education. Hearings: "Reauthorization of the Older Americans Act," Washington, D.C., February and March 1978.

U.S. House of Representatives. Hearings: "Second Supplemental Appropriation Bill, 1976—Part 1," Washington, D.C., 1976.

U.S. House of Representatives, Select Committee on Aging. "Federal Responsibility to the Elderly: Executive Programs and Legislative Jurisdiction." Washington, D.C.: U.S. Government Printing Office, 1977a.

U.S. House of Representatives, Select Committee on Aging. Hearings: "Fragmentation of Services for the Elderly," Washington, D.C., April 4, 1977. Washington, D.C.: U.S. Government Printing Office, 1977b.

U.S. House of Representatives, Select Committee on Aging. Hearings: "Reauthorization of the Older Americans Act: A Case For a Complete Overhaul," August 1977c.

U.S. House of Representatives, Select Committee on Aging, Subcommittee on Housing and Consumer Interests. Hearings: "Older Americans Act: Impact on the Minority Elderly," Los Angeles, Calif., August 23, 1977d.

U.S. House of Representatives, Select Committee on Aging. Hearings: "Older Americans Programs Oversight," August 3, September 15, 1977. Washington, D.C.: U.S. Government Printing Office, 1977e.

U.S. House of Representatives, Select Committee on Aging, Subcommittee on Federal, State, and Community Services. Hearings: "Title XX Social Services and the Elderly," Washington, D.C., October 27, 1977f.

U.S. House of Representatives, Select Committee on Aging. Hearings: "Older Americans Programs Oversight," March 1978a.

U.S. House of Representatives, Select Committee on Aging. Hearings: "Older Americans Act Reauthorization," March 2, 1978b.

U.S. House of Representatives, Select Committee on Aging. Hearings: "Older Americans Programs Oversight," Chester, Pa., March 3, 1978c.

U.S. House of Representatives, Select Committee on Aging. "Area Agencies on Aging and the Older Americans Act." Washington, D.C.: U.S. House of Representatives, March 17, 1978d.

U.S. House of Representatives, Select Committee on Aging. "Poverty among America's Aged." Unpublished staff review, August 8, 1978e.

U.S. House of Representatives, Select Committee on Aging. Hearings, Cincinnati, Ohio, August 21, 1978f.

U.S. House of Representatives. "Comprehensive Older Americans Act Amendments of 1978," Report No. 95–1618, September 22, 1978.

U.S. Senate, Special Committee on Aging. Hearings: "Trends in Long-Term Care," October 14, 28, 1971. Washington, D.C.: U.S. Government Printing Office, 1971.

U.S. Senate, Committee on Government Operations, Subcommittee on Intergovernmental Relations. Hearings, 1973.

U.S. Senate, Special Committee on Aging. *Developments in Aging: 1975 and January–May 1976.* Report No. 94–998, Part I. Washington, D.C.: U.S. Government Printing Office, 1976a.

U.S. Senate, Special Committee on Aging, Subcommittees on Long-Term Care and on Health of the Elderly. Joint hearings: "Medicare and Medicaid Frauds," Washington, D.C., 1975–1976. Washington, D.C.: U.S. Government Printing Office, 1976b.

U.S. Senate, Special Committee on Aging. *Developments in Aging: 1976.* Report No. 95–88, Part I. Washington, D.C.: U.S. Government Printing Office, 1977.

U.S. Senate, Committee on Human Resources, Subcommittee on Aging. Hearings: "Oversight and Extension of the Older Americans Act," Washington, D.C., February 1978a.

U.S. Senate, Special Committee on Aging. *Developments in Aging: 1977.* Report No. 95–771, Part I. Washington, D.C.: U.S. Government Printing Office, 1978b.

Van Til, J., and Van Til, S. "Citizen Participation in Social Policy: The End of the Cycle?" *Social Problems,* 1970, *17,* 313–323.

Veterans Administration. *Annual Report: Administration of Veterans Affairs.* Washington, D.C.: U.S. Government Printing Office, 1977.

Waldhorn, S. A., and others. "Planning and Participation: General Revenue Sharing in Ten Large Cities." Menlo Park, Calif.: Stanford Research Institute, 1975.

Walker, A. "Poverty in Old Age and the Social Creation of Dependency." Paper presented at the meeting of the International Sociological Association, Uppsala, Sweden, August 1978.

Warren, R. L. "Competing Objectives in Special Revenue Sharing." Paper presented at the Stanford Research Institute Conference on Approaches to Accountability in Postcategorical Programs, Menlo Park, Calif., August 1973a.

Warren, R. L. "Comprehensive Planning and Coordination: Some Functional Aspects." *Social Problems,* 1973b, *20,* 355–364.

Warren, R. L., Rose, S. M., and Bergunder, A. F. *The Structure of Urban Reform.* Lexington, Mass.: Lexington Books, 1974.

Weber, M. "Bureaucracy." In H. H. Gerth and C. W. Mills (Trans. and Eds.), *From Max Weber: Essays in Sociology.* New York: Oxford University Press, 1946. (Originally published 1922.)

Westat, Inc. *Evaluation of the Area Planning and Social Services Program (July 1974–June 1976).* Vol. 1: *Focus on Changes in Services to Older Persons: The Area Agency Role.* Prepared for Administration on Aging. Rockville, Md.: Westat, Inc., 1978a.

Westat, Inc. *Evaluation of the Area Planning and Social Services Program (July 1974–June 1976).* Vol. 2: *Program Description.* Prepared for Administration on Aging. Rockville, Md.: Westat, Inc., 1978b.

Zander, M. "Welfare Reform and the Urban Aged." *Transaction Society,* 1978, *15,* 59–66.

Zorn, F. E., Rose, L., and Radin, B. "Title XX and Public Participation: An Overview." *Public Welfare,* 1976, *34* (4), 20–25.
Zucker, L. G., and Estes, C. L. "Research Proposal to Study Revenue Sharing and Aging." Los Angeles: Institute for Social Science Research, University of California, 1976.

Index